Praise for Mary Michele McCarville's

American Doctor

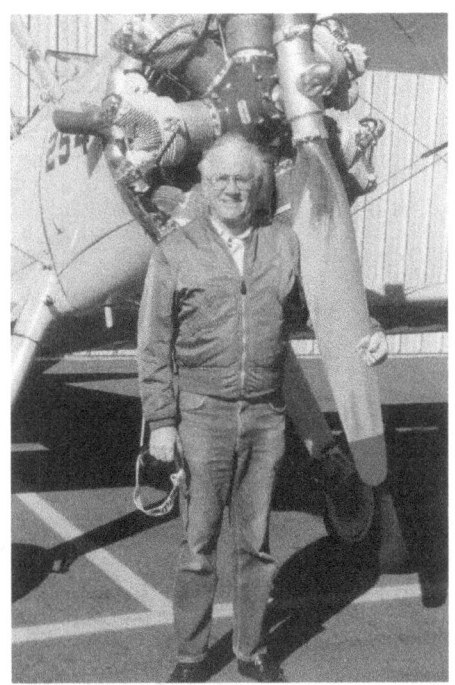

"American Doctor is at once intimate and comprehensive in scope. Not only do we learn about a unique and compassionate physician who survived many obstacles to reach his goal, but we are privy to a slice of Irish history that serves to acquaint us with the common struggles of the Irish immigration to America. We discover the ancestors of John McCarville--going back to 1848- faced with the excruciating decision of remaining in an impoverished and tyrannical land or making a precarious voyage with the entire family to a new life. Fortunately for the author, who is the daughter of the "American Doctor," the latter was chosen. We are given a bird's-eye view of the harshness of sea travel at that time as well as the reality of life in Ireland under English rule. Once the immigrants landed in New York, many more tribulations lay ahead for the McCarville family. However, their fortitude and religious convictions overcame many of them. Throughout this journey, the author conveys a strong sense of pride in her family origins and reveals their foibles, which add to the authenticity of the saga. Jack McCarville is certainly an inherent part of early Arizona history. From the moment he left his native state of Iowa to settle in the little known Sonoran Desert, he made his mark in what is now known as "The Valley of the Sun." We are told of his struggling days in medical school, the time and energy it took to build a practice, the medical procedures that he took upon himself to perfect and the eventual change in our country's healthcare system. Yet, Jack always seemed to have a quest for learning that went into such disparate fields as aviation and ballroom dancing. His love of life certainly is evident in his love for his family as well as for his fellow man. This biography by a very devoted daughter pays loving homage to a very special human being."

-Honey Levin

"I am finding this is a great book, especially the first chapter about the immigration. The descriptions are the most graphic and detailed I have seen of the trip from Ireland to the USA by our ancestors. The author has written so well and clear, I felt (nearly) that I was a passenger on the Chaos; I must confess that at one point I was brought to weeping over the tragedy of the Irish immigration and the plight of getting to U.S. soil. I have also enjoyed the other chapters, and the details of the life and accomplishments of Dr. McCarville. He obviously is a man of great vision, and has enjoyed and reached many horizons. His love and regard for his fellow man and the people he comes in contact with, along with his other attributes, sets him apart from most of us".

-Julian Smith

One pilot Jack sees on a regular basis, airline pilot James Medlock described Jack to his daughter Michelle in accurate detail. His email to her follows. "I first began seeing your Dad seven years ago for my FAA physicals. I admired his quick wit and great sense of humor the very first visit, and look forward to my yearly visits to his office to hear about his latest escapade, or the current topic of his latest concern for our country. He truly is a great man of the old school. He values people, he is unselfish, his word is his life, and he knows all about hard work and the struggles of life for the common man. I think that is why he can relate so well with people. He doesn't see $$ signs, he sees inside to our spirit. He is a very uplifting and positive individual and always lifts the spirit of all who come into contact with him. I learned a great deal about his concerns for America's health care system. A topic he and I have discussed many times, as well as his determination and perseverance to gain his medical credentials. I think there should be great interest in his story at both the AMA and the Historical Society of Phoenix. He is a physician icon in the "Valley of the Sun".

-James Medlock
–Captain US Airway
(Retired)

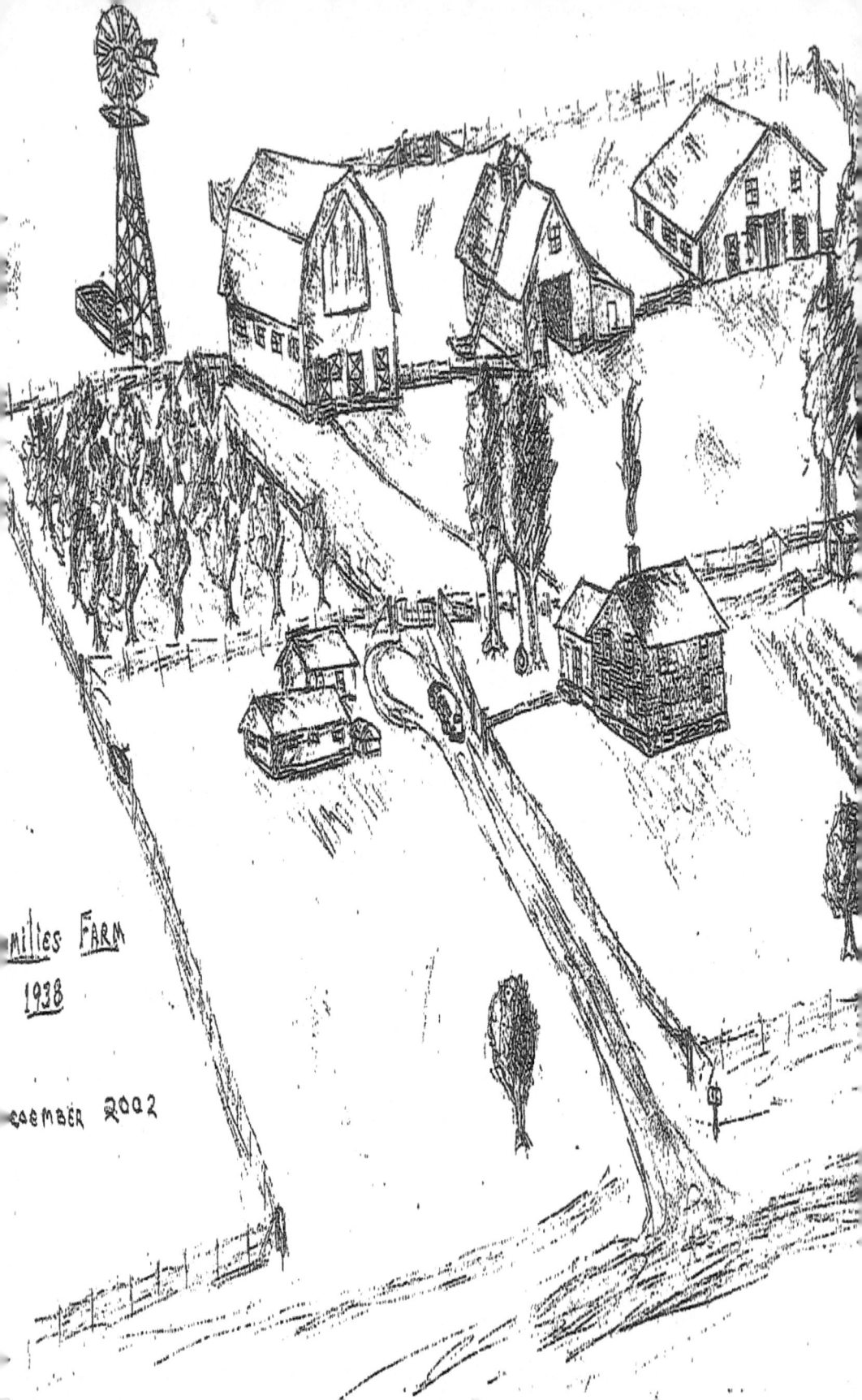

American Doctor

Aviation Medical Examiner

Michele, Your father has been my flight surgeon for most of the last two decades. He ended up becoming far more than simply a doctor. Your dad's extensive knowledge of the human condition and human psyche allowed him to answer every question and solve every dilemma that I presented to him. None of these inquires were especially unusual or uncommon, but all were important to this aviator when he was a new hire airline pilot in his early twenties. His advice was equally important during my early thirties as a new Captain. Today, easing into middle age, Dr. McCarville's advice and guidance are as important as ever. What makes this remarkable, is the fact that many, if not most, of your dad's patients feel the same way. Though much of this information is medical in nature, your dad provides a vital part of the health care for thousands of aviation professionals. After a recent medical examination by your dad he told me about the book that you wrote titled American Doctor. Not being able to buy his copy I ordered one from Amazon that same day. After the package was received, I sat down with American Doctor and read it cover to cover, finally sleeping in the small hours of the morning. By itself, your book is outstanding. Your ability to weave history into a biography in an interesting fashion is unusual. Few authors have your skills. Of particular interest was your research into the early family years in Ireland and the politics of Ireland and England and the resulting immigration to the United States. These days, the stories of the European immigrations are all but forgotten. Your book reminds us that this was not so long ago. The McCarville history in the Catholic Church was my favorite part of your book. I must admit that American Doctor serves well as a manual on the Catholic religion for this Lutheran husband. I gave a copy of American Doctor to my father and he appreciated the paragraphs of your dad treating Medal of Honor Ira Hays. Learning of your dad's volunteerism was no surprise. Some of the sad parts of your book moved me to tears. Great writers make an emotional impact on their readers. I look forward to my next physical and your next book. Captain John Bergeson, US Airways.

By

Mary Michele McCarville

for

Jack

and

the angels who follow him

Acknowledgments

Thanks to Don Rose, Gordy McCarville and Jim McCarville for the McCarville website, especially to Jim who encouraged me personally on this book. Special credits to members of the McCarville website for any material or photographs.

Thanks to Steve McCarville for editing and sketch.

Thanks to Sister Virginia McCarville, FSPA for historical material, pictures, editing, guidance and prayers. Every letter and email from Sister Virginia is reflected in this book. My father and I found proof through her, angels do exist.

Thanks to Jim Medlock, Captain US Airways (retired) for his verification of the importance of writing this biography.

Thanks loving thanks to my husband, I am his number one.

Thanks loving thanks to my children Tommy, Rachel and my mother for her contributions, and family members and friends involved in providing material and editing suggestions.

Thanks to Honey Levin for editing and her reference to Barbara Burke for promotion to the Irish Cultural Center in Phoenix, Arizona.

Special loving thanks to my father for his patience with the endless interviews, phone calls, faxes and editing. He has and always will be an inspiration to me.

Contents

	Page
Acknowledgements..................................	9
Introduction...	12
Chapter One...	16
A. Farewell to Shamrock	
Chapter Two..	45
A. New York, Wisconsin	
Chapter Three..	64
A. Iowa	
Chapter Four	118
A. Arizona General Practice, Family Life	
Chapter Five..	169
A. Aviation Medicine	
About the Author.....................................	220

Introduction

John Edward McCarville, fondly called Jack, grew up on a farm in Moorland, Iowa. He was the second child of an Irish Catholic family of eight. Frail and stricken with asthma, he traveled to Arizona alone at the age of 17 for his respiratory health. He set upon his goal to become a doctor and attended premedical classes at a college in Tempe, Arizona now known as Arizona State University (ASU). After discharge from the U.S. Army, he went on to obtain a degree in medicine from Creighton University in Omaha, Nebraska in 1951.

Jack married and moved back to Phoenix, Arizona where he set up a general practice in 1953 next to an old-fashioned soda fountain pharmacy. He ran a successful practice for years before the advent of managed care. He warned the nation of the dangers of suffocation from plastic bags, became a pilot, was flight surgeon for the Arizona Army National Guard and examined a 9/11 terrorist.

Major changes in the health care insurance industry propelled him from family practice into aviation medicine full time. Still in practice today, he is one of the few First Class FAA Medical Examiners in the state of Arizona. This biography provides an intricate detailed background of his Irish Catholic heritage and his life experiences with the evolution of medical care, insurance, technology and the market force dynamics of the healthcare industry from the depression era until present day.

Exodus 23:20

Behold, I send an Angel before thee, to keep thee in the way, and to bring thee into the place which I have prepared.

Chapter One

When John Edward McCarville, fondly called Jack, was a 10 year old boy in Moorland, Iowa he knew he was Irish when he heard his father talk about his great great grandfather Dennis Daniel McCarville. Dennis Daniel was one of the million citizens from Ireland who sailed 3,000 miles across the Atlantic Ocean in the first mass migration to America. In 1848 Dennis Daniel who was born in 1782, agonized about the trek his wife Mary, 13 year old son Dennis Michael , 20 year old niece Mary and 19 year old daughter Bridget (known as Biddy) were about to take. Dennis Daniel and Mary Cassady married in 1815 and had six children, five sons and one daughter. Dennis Daniel purchased embarkation tickets for a family of five at three pounds each. They were to sail from the Waterloo Dock at Liverpool to New York on a new 771 ton vessel built in 1847 named the Chaos. A strong male must travel with a family on such voyages as lines for daily cooking on the ship are long and prone to shoving and fighting. The tickets Dennis Daniel purchased were for a small berth with four bunk beds; Mary and Biddy will sleep together on one of the beds. The word steerage means third class accommodations during travel on a ship, and is not much better than what livestock must endure. Steerage fare on the Chaos required passengers to bring their own sheets, pillows and food provisions as only rations of bread, water, and cooking wood was included in the price of the tickets.

Dennis Daniel and his family packed one change of clothing to avoid carrying too much weight during their walk to the ferry at Belfast. The type of clothing Irish peasants wore at this time consisted of woolens and corduroy for men and linens and cotton for women. Thomas, the very elderly father of Dennis Daniel was responsible for filling five heavy large bags, one for each family member to carry over their shoulder for food supplies for three months. The food supply consisted of large amounts of dried meat and fish, flour, flatbread, cheese, dried peas, butter, onions, oatmeal, a keg of thin milk, tea, salt, pepper, a cooking pot, dishes and eating utensils. A laying chicken struggled in a wooden crate to provide the family eggs and a chicken dinner if necessary. Dennis Daniel planned to cook oatmeal for breakfast and a daily dinner stew on the upper deck of the ship over a fire built on a sand pit in the ships galley. He would have to balance himself while cooking during rough seas, and in severe weather, his family would eat cheese and flatbread.

Even though the elderly Thomas was frail, he was over six foot tall. He struggled not to weep as he looked at his son Dennis Daniel with his brilliant blue eyes. He would mourn for him for the rest of his life, as he was too old to sail to America. So many Irish peasants said good-bye this way to their loved ones that the tragedy became known as the American Wake. Thomas reassured Dennis he would care for his remaining four sons until he could send money for their passage on another ship. The majority of McCarville descendants are very tall and having longevity- many reach well into their 90's. The oldest recorded McCarville was 107 years old! Jack's family tree starts with Thomas McCarville (I), born in 1720 in County Monaghan. Thomas (I) had five boys, but the exact name of his wife remains unknown. This particular couple accounts for over 75% of the McCarville descendants now numbering well over 23,000. Thomas (I) named his third son after himself, an Irish tradition during the time, he was born in 1750 in Clones. This son is Thomas (II) who had two wives; his first wife was Mary Codden. She had five children with Thomas (II); their first child was a son, Dennis Daniel. Mary Codden died during the Irish Rebellion of 1798. After her death, Thomas (II) married Jane McGuire. She helped care for Dennis Daniel and the other children on an 8-acre potato farm in Western County Monaghan in the Northern Province of Ulster. Jane McGuire had two children with Thomas (II) - he had seven children in all- Dennis Daniel, Felix, Philip, Patrick, Bridget, Thomas and Michael.

Ancient history regarding the name of McCarville in Ireland reveals the initial name to be "Son of Carroll". The Carroll's descend from Caerbhaill (pronounced Karvel in Gaelic) meaning "fierce in battle." The Caerbhaill were kings of the Oriel province ruling five counties to include Monaghan from 950 AD. During the Norman invasion, two Norman princes were battling for land and the Caerbhaill king at the time was Muircheartach O'Carroll. He found himself in the middle of a huge battle between the two Norman princes but unfortunately chose the wrong side. Muircheartach O'Carroll was hanged in 1194 after being brutally blinded during his capture.

In 1848, Thomas (II) McCarville, Mary Coddan and the children lived in the parish of Aghabog, which centered on Saint Mary's Church built in 1820. Irish peasants grouped together in clans made up of a few family names who dominated a parish. Each clan formed a town made up of about 40 families on a few hundred acres. Families lived in three room houses with walls made of sun dried mud two feet thick supported by timber. All the houses were high enough for a man of six foot three to stand in; they were partially underground and blended in with the landscape. Floors were dirt, packed down hard but in wet weather became muddy; roofs were thatched with straw.

The inside of the three rooms of the McCarville home was primitive in construction. One room was where the family all slept with each bed having four posts and a canopy to prevent bugs from the roof falling on the bed. Ireland had rain every day but with hard rain, brown water dripped down and small animals such as a mouse plunked through the straw. The largest room had a three-legged wooden stool next to a huge kettle hanging over a fire pit. The family lived on root vegetables and milk. Fuel was peat moss collected from the bogs. There was no chimney so smoke would filter out through holes in the thatched roof or sometimes out the door or lone window. The most important room for survival was the third room. This was for livestock which was sometimes necessary in order to pay the monthly rent to the local English deputy. If the rent became late the family would face eviction.

The Irish did not pay in coin so the English deputies collected grain, produce, meat, flax, woven linen and livestock from the peasants every month. The deputy forwarded the proceeds to the Belfast ferry to Liverpool to be distributed to various English proprietors. Thomas and Dennis Daniel grew flax on their land for the linen trade; an industry introduced to Ireland by the Phoenicians before Christ was born. Both men met often with the Irish merchants who traveled to Belfast. Some were able to smuggle back newspapers from the Northern Star. After one family read the newspaper, the paper was passed on to another family. Over 50 families would read one single newspaper. Most of the articles were encouraging the Irish to rebel against the English, the newspaper was banned in 1793.

If a deputy evicted a family of peasants, they "papered" the door of the house with an eviction notice three weeks prior; then English soldiers tore or burned the house down to prevent them from moving back. English property owners favored eviction as they were interested in reorganizing the farmlands into larger sections. Evicted families were forced to move to a workhouse to keep a roof over their heads, but some went to prison or worse if they fought eviction. English soldiers murdered resistant peasants and houses were often searched for no reason. The houses of the native Irish were easy for the English to tear down; but in every family community, two houses were often made of stone - one for the priest and the other for a school for the children. The poorest peasants relied solely on potato crops, could not read, write or speak English. As they had no other trade or livestock, they would often be late with their rent. Thomas (II) and his family learned to speak English and were able to survive with their trades in farming, butchering and the linen weaving business.

England obtained Ireland by military control and the rents Her Majesty charged eventually reduced the majority of the native Irish to poverty. The English regarded Irish natives with disgust and fools they called Paddy. The Paddy was viewed as a lazy, rebellious people who grew the simple lowly potato, enjoyed living in poverty with pigs in mud houses and dressing in rags. The proprietor for Dennis Daniel and Thomas was an Englishman named Lord Rossmore who owned the majority of the land in the area but did not care what happened to the local peasants. Although the majority of the Irish soon learned English, they remained resistant to the Protestant Church of Ireland. They continued to practice their Catholic faith in secret. Each town land took care of their local priest and provided him with food and a well-built house.

When the native Irish lost their churches to the English and were discouraged from the practice of their Catholic religion, they met in a different field every week for Mass. The McCarville clan often met at the Mass Rock, which was a nearby ancient tomb that had enormous rocks forming a structure. Ireland is famous for ancient tombs. The concept of fairies in Irish folklore relates to how the dead live on in tiny beautiful towns within these ancient burial chambers. The McCarvilles used flatbread and a simple cup for the Sacrament of Communion on a flat portion of the Mass Rock. If the English "redcoats" came near, the younger Irish standing guard at the nearest crossroad would begin dancing in furious hard stomps to the music of the violin or bagpipe to warn those who were attending Mass. During Christmas, care was taken for the location of the celebration of Mass so as not to be discovered. Midnight Mass out of necessity was said on Christmas Eve in a designated barn in every town land. A single candle would be placed at dusk in the window of the barn where Mass was to be said in secret. In the winter, most windows were packed with greenery to keep the cold out; the appearance of a wreath with a lone candle was created. After everyone in the town knew whose barn to make their way to in the middle of the night for midnight Mass on Christmas Eve, they put a candle in their own windows to confuse the English soldiers of the location.

The Irish view education as a priority for children and will sacrifice to donate to a school and teacher in every township. Children would sit on a dirt floor, most in bare feet, and listen to a teacher who might also be bare footed. Children learned the importance of Irish tradition: family values, religion and culture. Language was Gaelic. Story time was Irish folklore, stories about the sea and mystical relationships to the land they loved, respected and lived in. Every child knew the intense stubborn resistance their parents had toward the rules of the English. The English found the

Irish may have been easy to conquer, but were very difficult to rule!

Thomas (II) had worked hard all his life for his family but now he was packing them up to leave Ireland, encouraging them to go on a dangerous voyage, which could possibly end their lives. Dennis Daniel was unable to look back to his father when they started the long walk to the Belfast ferry for the port of Liverpool. The town priest came to the house to bless Dennis Daniel and other families that were leaving. Many tears were shed. Even though the English knew the peasants were starving from the famine, the English distributed no emergency food supplies to them. All the produce of Ireland the English collected from the peasants went to Liverpool.

Dennis Daniel was curious and excited to see the famous city of Liverpool. However, he was dreading the voyage. The voyage time to New York could range from 3 weeks to 3 months depending on the weather. He realized his family would have a long walk to the Belfast ferry and struggle with the weight of the food required for that length of time. Then at Liverpool, they may have to camp and wait for their ship for weeks at the Waterloo port. In addition, he heard this voyage to New York was very dangerous since the ships at the time were not regulated for safety.

When Dennis said his final good-bye to Thomas, he knew he would never return to Ireland or see him again. He grabbed his father with a physical convulsion of sorrow he had never known and sunk his face into his chest and sobbed uncontrollably. When they broke apart, they looked at each other one last time; they did not know what lie ahead for any of them. Dennis Daniel moved on to say goodbye to his four tall, strong sons. He had concern but felt confident he would see them again. He cautioned them with rules he had learned from his own father for survival. They must stay aware of danger, be humble and not take risks. He made them promise to protect each other and stay together when they traveled to

America after he sent money for passage. It would take Dennis Daniel less than a year to have his sons Thomas, Francis, Patrick and Joseph join him in New York. Soon after, his father passed away.

The potato famine started in 1845 by the fungus *Phytophthora infestans* which the Irish simply called "blight". This fungus was a known menace for potato crops grown mostly by the poor in Ireland. The soil and climate in Ireland is moist and ideal for growing the potato, but any fungus thrives in moisture. Irish peasants were usually able to produce enough potatoes to sustain their family on very small plots of land. On occasion, blight would affect crops but not to a severe degree. When blight occurs, a black rot develops around the leaves, stems and the soil surrounding the potato plant, disabling photosynthesis necessary for plant survival. In 1847, a severely cold winter prompted blight to overwhelm the majority of potato crops and the enormous suffering from starvation and disease became known as "Black 47". Peasants were forced to eat precious seed potatoes or use them to pay rent to avoid eviction, reducing the chances of future crops.

Dennis and Thomas kept the family alive with livestock, linen weaving and work as butchers for the English. However, the majority of the Irish were begging for food from soup kitchens run by the Quakers because the English plan was to ultimately starve the entire population. English workhouses kept Irish peasants of all age's working day and night sewing, weaving linen or performing hard labor. The starvation from famine caused so many deaths that the English had a serious health problem keeping up with disposing of the bodies. When babies lost their parents due to starvation, they were branded by the English. The English then paid wet nurses to feed the babies every month but usually the wet nurses would dispose of the babies after they collected their money. Soon the English realized that paying the peasants' passage to America would be cheaper than supporting them. Some peasants left for America after eviction with passages paid for by the

English and others left on their own when diseases such as cholera prompted emigration.

Dennis Daniel sought out stories about an older distant relative from a nearby town whose name was Thomas McCarville; he was one of the first McCarvilles to sail to America. He enlisted in the U.S. Army and served during the War of 1812. The army defended the attack and the burning of the U.S. Capitol by British troops who forced President James Madison and his wife Dolly to flee for their lives. The next attack against the U.S. Capitol would not be until September 11, 2001. Thomas left the army on November 26, 1816 and obtained 160 acres of bounty land in McDonough County, Illinois in 1818.

This idea of land ownership excited Dennis Daniel, as his family had been tenants to despicable British landowners for years. Dennis Daniel decided on the move to America with curious determination and chose New York for a new future for himself and his family. Most McCarville relatives immigrated to Prince Edward Island (PEI) and became successful potato farmers, growing a vast variety of potatoes. Dennis Daniel realized PEI could provide a safe haven for his family, but he was different from most men. His intense curiosity and sense of adventure drove him to decide on exposing himself and his family to the more dangerous risk of traveling to America.

When Dennis Daniel and his family boarded the ferry at Belfast after an exhausting walk, burdened with the heavy sacks they carried for survival, they collapsed and slept on the deck for over 10 hours before reaching the Waterloo Dock. When the ferry landed, they stood up in shock and awe at the change in their environment. They had come from beautiful countryside to the dirty, noisy city of Liverpool with crowds of oddly dressed people speaking strange languages among very tall, brick buildings. There was a smell of smoke, sewage and a roar of noise in all directions. Donkey carts were everywhere pulling people with their possessions stacked high. A mother of nine was shouting and crying as she tried to find two of her small children, who had been lost for hours. Large ships were docked in every inch of space with tall, white sails and rough talking sailors working hard to prepare for a voyage. Dennis hardly slept while protecting his family from vicious thieves while they camped near the Chaos for over a week. He was so exhausted when they boarded the ship 24 hours before sailing that he stumbled on the deck and fell on his food sack. While Mary was helping him up, they both turned in horror and watched a desperate ragged family of four attempting to board without tickets, screaming for mercy while being driven back down to the dock. Right before sailing, a boy of 12 years of age was found as a stowaway in a barrel full of biscuits. He was allowed to stay after a sympathetic man paid his fare.

The voyage on the Chaos was grueling due to winter weather; Dennis and the stronger passengers struggled to keep the heavy wooden hatch open for light and air as much as possible. Violent storms caused the ship to pitch and roll from side to side and lightning terrified everyone. Although the ship had wooden tables and benches attached to the floor, boxes and barrels would often become unsecured from their ropes and roll about. Fresh milk was lost in the middle of the voyage when a milk cow was thrust overboard in one extreme storm. During these storms, the stronger men climbed up the narrow wooden ladders and shut the large doors tight. The steerage passengers then had to deal with the pitch-darkness and stench of the miserably close quarters of the ship, already overcrowded with passengers who were seasick and not in the best of health. Even with the cold winter weather of December, the air in the lower deck soon became hot, humid and rancid. Passengers often suffered from panic and screamed out in misery.

Near the middle of the voyage on a cool, sunny day, Dennis Daniel enjoyed watching a sweet, playful girl of three on the upper deck. That night she had a high fever and severe vomiting which lasted for two days before she died. Her tiny body was covered in a bright red rash. When the captain saw her, he ordered her to be immediately wrapped in canvas and brought to the upper deck. After a short prayer, she was buried at sea with her trembling parents looking on in grief. Sharks gathered round, and the captain quickly moved her parents away before they could witness what was about to happen. The sharks never stopped following the ship after that. Most of the passengers buried at sea from "ship fever" or typhus were elderly or young. The ships on these voyages became known as "coffin ships" due to the many deaths at sea.

    Dennis Daniel had packed medicinal preparations and used water rations to mix with lye soap to clean the family bunk area on a daily basis. Each bunk was made from rough wood and stacked into a double deck bed. The mattresses were stuffed with straw and commonly infested with lice and fleas, which could prompt typhus. Dennis had his family fill the clothes they slept in at night with a sprig of rosemary and lavender to prevent fleabites. Between the four wooden bunks beds was a single stand with a metal basin they filled with water, using lye soap for a "spit bath." Individual towels hung up on a hook to dry and they used a lard candle for light. Dennis mixed a powder of arrowroot plant into a tea for his family to drink on a daily basis to prevent nausea and vomiting. Primitive toilet facilities were available on each side of the ship with long lines before reaching the wretched destination. The stench from the toilets or the seasickness blended with an odor of vinegar which was heated to emit steam in an attempt to purify the air. Dennis had family members wear a scarf scented with a mixture of eucalyptus oil and menthol over their face when waiting in line for the toilet.

One evening, an elderly Irish passenger Dennis had become fond of suddenly died. After he was buried at sea, Dennis knelt where his wife was sitting and cried in her lap, begging her to forgive him for what he had done to their family. Mary looked up in tears at their daughter Bridget, known as Biddy who was standing near the deck. Biddy drew close when she saw the pain in her mother's dark brown eyes. Biddy was called "Dot" by her parents, a common Irish nickname for a daughter. Although her brothers had fair skin, dark brown hair and brilliant blue eyes, Dot had the coloring called Black Irish, appearing to be of Spanish descent. She had an unusually fair white complexion, dark brown eyes with full black eyebrows, jet-black hair and was beautiful. Her father Dennis Daniel had jet-black hair as a boy but was prematurely grey by the age of 25, a genetic trait common in the Black Irish group.

Dot looked at her mother who appeared so fragile, saw her father suffering and began to sing. Dot sang a folksong of a fisherman encountering a dragon in the sea. Passengers from private cabins drew closer to hear her sing. After a moment an Irish man began to play a violin, then another a flute. When Dot finished singing, an Irish bagpipe began to play alone, full of sorrow as well as hope. Many descendants of the McCarville family have abilities in dance, sports, and music. On February 19, 2008, Jack's daughter Michelle, a fifth cousin to the mother of Calgary Flames Dion Phaneuf, sat on the glass cheering her relative on to win his fight against the Phoenix Coyotes. Another relative, Janel McCarville, a woman of six foot two inches tall from Wisconsin, has a career with the WNBA. The steerage passengers of the Chaos fell together at their first glimpse of land shouting with joy, dancing to the music of a violin. Dennis Daniel walked away from the frenzy and stood alone looking at the strange horizon of New York. He thought of an Irish poem by Tom Moore. "Erin! Oh! Erin, thy night it is past, and the sunshine of freedom dawns on thee at last."

Years later, Dennis Daniel refused to speak of this voyage to America and family members knew not to ask. The Chaos docked in New York in a port on the East River across from Brooklyn. There was no Statue of Liberty yet to welcome the family but New York was over 30% Irish. Immigration regulations at this time existed at each port of entry by individual states and officers reviewed the health of each arriving immigrant. Health concerns ranged from diphtheria, tuberculosis, measles and a contagious disease of the eye called trachoma they examined for by turning the eyelid over with a buttonhook. This eye disease was of particular concern as it could lead to blindness. In 1848, the average life expectancy for a person was 47 years old, 30% of deaths from infectious disease. The voyage on the Chaos was a dangerous battle for Dennis Daniel and his family but they were robust, and easily passed health inspections. They made verbal declarations of name, age, occupation, point of origin and ship name, all recorded in a hand written log that still exists today.

Later, in 1891, legislation passed for government officials to develop Ellis Island to control the massive influx of immigrants as the numbers had risen too high for individual states to process. This began the formation of the U.S. Public

Health Service to assess the health of immigrants arriving, sometimes in numbers reaching over 10,000 a day. Those who failed initial exams were admitted to a hospital or in severe cases sent back to their country of origin. Tickets purchased at this time were required to be round trip tickets. This was very profitable for the shipping business as none of the immigrant passengers wanted to make the return trip. Families were forced to leave ill loved ones behind in one of the 27 hospitals built on islands in New York created of fill, some patients stayed for years for tuberculosis treatment. Ellis Island became the Isle of Hope or, depending on the circumstances, for a family who left a patient behind in one of these hospitals, the Isle of Tears.

When Dennis Daniel McCarville set foot on American soil December 14, 1848, he was on a quest for his family's survival but had dreams of land ownership with fertile soil and a free government. Dennis Daniel and his family had been shocked at the city of Liverpool, but now faced an even more dramatic change in their environment when they reached New York. Their lives of poor farmers in the beautiful farmland of Ireland under the cruel rule of the English changed to Irish emigrants living in the busy, noisy city of New York. Instantly, their personal identity changed. They were not under English rule and could speak Irish if they wished. They would not starve here and most likely, would maintain their health. Dennis was happy to realize he and his family could finally practice their Roman Catholic religion in freedom. They would experience prejudice but were not in the midst of war.

      Dennis Daniel knew about war and discussed this issue with his sons before making the decision to go to New York. Dennis Daniel was only 13 years old when he joined his father and mother to fight the English in the Irish Rebellion at the Battle of Vinegar Hill in June of 1798. In this particular battle, an immense collection of 20,000 Irish men, women and children, many unarmed or only carrying a shovel, banded together and charged the English in desperation to gain back the rights they had lost to their land and religion. They were overcome after a valiant attempt, but when the Irish retreated, the English massacred men, women and children in hundreds as they ran for safety.

During this time, the majority of native Irish wore a shamrock or a string of green on their wrists, shoelaces or as a scarf to show their support of United Irishmen. The color green represents hope and the shamrock is a symbol of spring or rebirth. The United Irishmen were a republican revolutionary group often called "croppies" due to their short haircuts as an anti-wig protest statement against the English. In response, the English tortured United Irishmen rebels they captured with "pitch capping", pouring burning tar on their heads and ripping the skin off to deform them. Rebels that were found wearing the shamrock or "green" that the English captured were burned alive in their homes or hiding places and shot or hung in public.

Years later, the Irish recovered rights to make a living with a decrease in the Penal Laws of the English. However, their expertise in the linen weaving business soon brought competition between Irish Protestants and Irish Catholics in the same trade. A group of Irish Protestants known as the Orange tried to decrease the competition of the Catholics by destroying weaving machines in their homes in the early hours of the morning. These Protestants known as the "Peep of Day" boys were a serious problem in the area where Thomas and Dennis Daniel lived. Thomas and Dennis Daniel became part of a group known as the Green, also known as the "Defenders" to protect their clan from these early morning attacks by the Orange. The tricolor national flag of Ireland symbolizes a truce between these two groups by placing white as a symbol of peace between the colors of orange and green.

When Dennis Daniel arrived in New York, he joined many other men from Ireland who immediately dedicated themselves to their new country. Almost half of George

Washington's troops were of Irish descent. Dennis Daniel rented a one-room apartment near where the Twin Towers would later be built 1500 feet above the ground in 1971. The apartment building in 1848 was five stories high; apartments were available with one or two rooms, with mostly Irish living there. Plenty of jobs were available unloading, loading or building ships for six dollars a week. In addition, the lower east side of Manhattan had various factory jobs available especially in the clothing business.

After settling into their apartment, Dennis Daniel and Mary set out on a cold Christmas Eve to find food supplies to make a traditional Celtic seafood stew. They had to abstain from meat of flesh in order to receive Communion at Mass. In Ireland, traditionally on Christmas Eve, a piece of a dried salted fish called ling is cut up and served as a stew in fresh buttermilk with salt, pepper and parsley. Dennis Daniel and Mary were unable to find ling after searching in the New York market place and found the closest replacement was oysters.

Dennis Daniel heated thick round bowls, adding fresh butter to each bowl before pouring in shucked oysters, strained liquid from the oysters, fresh cream, butter, parsley, salt and pepper. Oyster stew became an Irish American tradition in most Irish families every Christmas Eve. Dennis Daniel served crisp buttered toast with the seafood stew as he chatted to Mary about her plum pudding in preparation with a goose they found at market to enjoy the next day, on Christmas Day, after Mass. As his family prayed before dinner, Dennis Daniel looked out the window of their small apartment at the snow in New York, on Christmas Eve. He rarely saw snow in Ireland. He realized he was home now and that he had a different flag to fly, to love, to fight and for which to die. This was his country, for himself and his family. Dennis Daniel laid his head down on the table, his big shoulders sobbing as he remembered his father clamoring, "They must be plucking the geese up in heaven!" whenever it snowed.

Chapter Two

Dennis Daniel and his family continued to live in New York with all four sons eventually sailing to America with money Dennis had sent back from his work in the shipping business. When his sons arrived they began working on the ships except for Thomas, he looked for work as a tailor. Thomas threw the newspaper down in a fury after reading the want ads where one stated, "Negros or Catholics need not apply." Mary and Biddy found work as domestic servants for a wealthy family in Manhattan and learned how to use a sewing machine. The lower east side of Manhattan had difficulty with various gangs of different ethnic groups. Irish gangs were called "Black Irish". The majority of people living in the area were foreign born with over 30% being Irish. The Irish harbored intense anger toward the English as they had fresh memories of the potato famine. This became evident in 1849 when a large group of Irish immigrants protested the Opera

Astor House when an English actor named Macready was in the play Macbeth. His first attempt at performing resulted in eggs and potatoes thrown on stage. When he was to perform on May 10, 1849 - a crowd of 20,000 people collected in front of the Astor House. A riot began with shots fired from the police directly into the crowd, killing 18 and wounding 40.

    Dennis Daniel and his family attended Mass on Sunday's at Saint Patrick's Old Cathedral on Mulberry Street in Manhattan. After Mass, Mary and Biddy always prepared a chicken dinner and Dennis Daniel relaxed reading the newspaper. He was especially interested to read about Irish Catholics settling in Wisconsin. Most of the information Dennis Daniel gathered indicated Wisconsin was similar to Ireland. Dennis studied the articles and soon became intent on joining the large community of Irish Catholics living there. However, most importantly, he wanted to buy his own land.

No one realized how many Irish Catholics lived in Wisconsin until Saint Patrick's Day, March 17, 1843 in Milwaukee. A crowd of over 3,000 Irish from numerous parishes organized together. Bishop Henni assigned Pastor Kundig to be in charge of the celebration at Saint Peter's Church in Milwaukee. He built a temporary altar in front of the church and had the German Milwaukee Band begin to play at four in the morning. A cannon was then shot off and the church bell rang for Mass to begin. At noon, an enormous collection of people started a procession with the grand marshal and his baton followed by the band. The choir of Saint Peter's Church and the large congregation followed singing as they displayed a huge banner of blue satin with three gilt stars in a wreath of shamrocks that read, "Education is the Road to Virtue." Because of the severe winter that year, snow forced everyone to be on foot or to be pulled in sleighs by horses. Different parishes in the area represented themselves with special personalized banners. Most banners combined the

American eagle with an Irish symbol, such as a shamrock in the bill of the eagle or the eagle hovering over an Irish harp. Examples of mottos on the banners were "Where Liberty Dwells There is My Country" and "Erin Go Bragh." This crowd was so overwhelming that Catholic bishops informed the Pope in Rome. After the report, the Pope approved the creation of a diocese naming Bishop Henni who was from Germany, as the first bishop in the Milwaukee diocese.

A few years after Dennis Daniel made his voyage to New York, German Catholics fled to America from Germany due to religious persecution. Nuns left when they were not allowed to wear their habits. Many Germans settled in Milwaukee along with the Irish. One group of Germans who would make an impact on the McCarville family was a small group of two priests and six nuns recruited by Bishop Henni of Wisconsin. This religious group was dedicated to the spirit of St. Francis of Assisi who lived in Italy from 1181 until 1226. The nuns Bishop Henni recruited intended to find a convent to teach children of immigrants and care for the sick. Bishop Henni helped the nuns purchase 53 acres five miles south of Milwaukee on Lake Michigan to build a convent following European rules of St. Francis. They wore a black habit, black cape with white turn over collar, black leather belt and a Franciscan cord under the habit. Their headdress was a white hood with a lace frill. The nuns taught in a school, cared for children in an orphanage and helped cut down trees to build their convent. The two German Catholic priests said Mass in a nearby parish church for the Sisters, where they practiced nocturnal adoration of the Blessed Sacrament following the rules of religious life in European convents. This rule follows the custom of the Sacrament being adored around the clock, every hour and minute of the day. In 1851, cholera or "yellow fever" was rampant and both priests suddenly died. The Sisters had no spiritual guides.

Bishop Henni stepped in and sent a number of priests to purchase land near the convent of the Sisters to build a seminary. The priests had the Sisters cook, clean, launder and garden for the seminary to save money. Initially, the Sisters felt this would be an advantage due to their location near priests. More importantly, they could restart nocturnal adoration of the Blessed Sacrament. However, the Sisters found they were unable to perform their duties to St. Francis of Assisi. The high demand of work to maintain the living quarters of the seminary disabled them from their goal of nocturnal adoration, teaching children or caring for the sick. One morning, they found themselves on the floor in a heap of exhaustion, still on their knees from evening prayers next to their beds. They were able to keep the seminary in excellent order but struggled to attend Mass or perform nocturnal adoration due to time limitations.

That afternoon, people in town watched the Sisters march to the post office where they mailed a letter to Bavaria requesting transfer back to Germany. Incredibly, they had requested to leave the safe haven of America and return to the religious persecution of Germany in order to improve the practice of their faith. They were in anxious anticipation when they received a letter back. The letter was on official letterhead signed and sealed by the top authority in charge of their order- stating refusal of admittance to the convent. The reason given was due to their ages as being too advanced. The Sisters shook with rage and disbelief when they read the letter. They were rejected as too old for their profession to God! They had no support or protection and were in a strange country. All they could do was pray.

Later that year a woman became aware about the plight of the Sisters from her spiritual director Father Heiss and applied to enter their convent. When she arrived, the German Sisters were certain she had come to them because of their prayers. This woman had a secret of shame, she had been married and divorced from an alcoholic husband and was using the maiden name of her mother to avoid discovery of her past. Although the Sisters were unaware of her history they knew immediately, she had a fierce nature and the ability to defend their convent. It did not take too many years for her to be chosen as Reverend Mother. Known as Mother Antonia Herb, she lived from 1827 until 1882, and was instrumental in leading the Sisters away from the workload at the seminary to a farm in Jefferson and then their final home, the Saint Rose Convent, in La Crosse, Wisconsin. The following article written by one of the Sisters at the St. Rose Convent details the history of events.

"Mother Antonia set to work immediately toward implementing the objectives of the early founders, to prepare the Sisters to teach in parochial schools. In order to do this, she knew she must secure a Motherhouse apart from and independent of all seminary control. The quest for an independent Motherhouse led to Jefferson, Wisconsin. It ended at a farmhouse near Saint Lawrence Church, two miles from the small town. Despite some objectives to the location, Mother Antonia and six Sisters came to Jefferson to take possession of that property on September 29, 1864. On that day, Saint Francis Convent, Milwaukee quietly yielded the title of Motherhouse to the little farm house, now to be called Saint Colleta Convent. The Jefferson years, 1864-1871 can be called the stabilization period of the struggling Franciscan Sisterhood. When the Eucharistic orientation was given its indelible seal and direction, when during its darkest days of 1865, Mother Antonia solemnly pledged that if God would bless the Community with stability, the Sisters would introduce perpetual adoration of the Eucharist, and in time, erect as beautiful a chapel to enshrine it, as means would allow. God heard the Sister's prayers.

Force of circumstances rather than freedom of choice and suitability had largely determined both the transfer of the Motherhouse to Jefferson and the exact site for the Colleta Convent. By the late 1860's it was evident that Jefferson with its inadequate transportation facilities and its limited cultural, education and healthcare opportunities was not an appropriate location. This time circumstances precipitated developments. La Crosse had opened as a new diocese. Father Heiss, who had been the spiritual director of the Sisters since 1852, was named the first bishop of La Crosse. It was logical that both Bishop Heiss and Mother Antonia should consider moving the Community's headquarters to La Crosse. In the summer of 1870, the cornerstone of Saint Rose Convent was laid. In July, 1871, St. Coletta Convent yielded its title."

The Sisters of the Saint Rose Convent consider a chapel a sacred place to allow guidance and inspiration within the quiet of prayer. Here they petition God to provide world peace, healing and blessings among a burning light to indicate a bright future. Mother Antonia died, but her promise was fulfilled. A clock was placed in the small chapel in the Saint Rose Convent to chime every hour and has done so since August 1, 1878. Since eleven in the morning on that day, at least two persons have prayed in the presence of the Blessed Sacrament around the clock for the city of La Crosse, the congregation, the Church and the world. The Franciscan Sisters of Perpetual Adoration, known as FSPA, established night and day adoration with the Blessed Sacrament exposed. In 1906, the Chapels of Mary of the Angels and of Perpetual Adoration was completed after four years. These chapels are named after a small church in Assisi, Italy given to Francis of Assisi. He named his chapel Maria Angelorum, as he believed he heard the songs of the angels there. The chapels in La Crosse have over 160 angels and 3 altars.

Dennis Daniel and his family continued to live in New York but dreamed of owning land in the countryside. In 1860, the family joined a crowd of over 1500 people at the Cooper Union Grand Hall in lower Manhattan to attend a speech against slavery given by a interesting lawyer from Illinois named Abraham Lincoln. The Cooper Union was a school offering classes in science and art that anyone could attend and had night classes for adults, which Dennis Daniel and his family enjoyed. In 1861, the Civil War broke out. The two

McCarville soldiers that are listed as serving in the Union Army in the Civil War indicate they were born in County Monaghan, Ireland and were from Wisconsin. The two sons of Dennis Daniel that were soon to serve were Francis and Thomas. They were privates in the 49 Wisconsin Infantry Company C.

Dennis Daniel exchanged letters with other McCarville relatives that settled in Wisconsin. When Dennis Daniel had enough money saved, he moved the entire family from New York to the town of Darlington, Wisconsin in November of 1862. They lived with other relatives in Darlington for a short time until Dennis Daniel purchased 120 acres of land. Dennis Daniel, Mary and their children thought they were walking back into Ireland. This land has beautiful rolling green hillsides near lakes to fish from and huge lush trees. Wild grape vines grow up high up in the trees with clusters of grapes hanging down. Wild blackberries and raspberries are everywhere. Black bears are in the area but are not aggressive. Dennis Daniel had heard stories from the older settlers in the area that they shot the bears for meat and were impressed with the taste of bear steaks. One old settler warned the family to be careful of vicious wildcats in the area as they could cause harm to the farm animals.

Dennis Daniel looked over the land before purchase as he wanted to build his family a house of stone and had seen enough in the area. He was happy the nearby town of Darlington already had the railroad, a store and school. In addition, there was a three-story hotel, courthouse, carpenter shop, blacksmith and sawmill. The diversity of immigrants in the town allowed many to become experts in their professions. For example, the Bohemians were known for shoemaking, Norwegians for wagon making and the Irish were experts in laundress.

When Dennis Daniel and his family moved to their land, they began to develop a dairy farm and collect stone to build a home. They soon realized they had purchased land suitable to start a stone quarry business. This land was rich in limestone called lannon stone, in high demand in the construction business. With dairy farming and the stone quarry, Dennis Daniel was able to purchase an additional 120 acres of land near Willow Springs, a total of 240 acres.

The lifelong dream of Dennis Daniel came true when he built his family a beautiful two story stone house on an incline in dense woods on the southeast corner of section four in Willow Springs, in Lafayette County on O'Neil road. This home is near Otter's Creek where deer run through and a spring close to the house supplies pure cold water among beautiful flowers and greenery. The stone house has a long wooden staircase and large basement that held Mary's enormous collection of colorful canned goods. Mary wanted sunlight filling the home so Dennis Daniel placed five large windows on each side of the house. He made two pentagon windows of lead and green glass and placed one on each end of the house, underneath the chimneys. The basement had small windows and was accessible only from the inside. He built two large fireplaces, one on each end. Three huge wooden doors enabled entry into the house, the extra door on the left side led to a summer kitchen. Dennis Daniel built a porch in the front where the family spent many evenings enjoying the sunsets. Mary was famous for her incredible gardens that included a vast variety of flowers and vegetables. She also planted various fruit trees and black walnut trees. Her favorite time was in the fall, when she could show off huge pumpkins she had grown for the county fair.

The family attended Mass every Sunday at the Holy Assumption Catholic Church. When Mary died in 1869, Dennis Daniel lived in the home with his son Dennis Michael and his family. He was still healthy in mind and body until one day while climbing up the worn staircase, which had sunk in the middle; he stopped and looked up at the sun coming through the window. For some unknown reason, he fell completely backwards down the stairs. Even at 99 years old, he was so strong that he lived for a week, dying with his third son Dennis Michael McCarville at his bedside on October 15, 1883. Dennis Daniel had named his son Dennis Michael following the Irish custom of naming the first name of your third son after yourself. At his funeral, Dennis Michael stood up to speak regarding his father as a "devoted Catholic, exemplary in his habits, a good citizen and a kind and indulgent father". Dennis Daniel is buried next to his wife Mary and their son Thomas, who had died previously at the early age of 49 years, at the Holy Assumption Cemetery in Willow Springs, Wisconsin.

The 240 acres of land for dairy farming and the stone quarry business had provided a steady income to Dennis Daniel and his family. The beautiful stone from the quarry was popular for paving, building, flagstone and curbs. Dennis Michael McCarville married Catherine Timmen, a girl whose parents had emigrated from Ireland and settled in Michigan, on April 13, 1864 in Mineral Point, Wisconsin. He never intended on moving from the beautiful stone home he had helped build and live in with his father and family. The home (below) still stands in 2009.

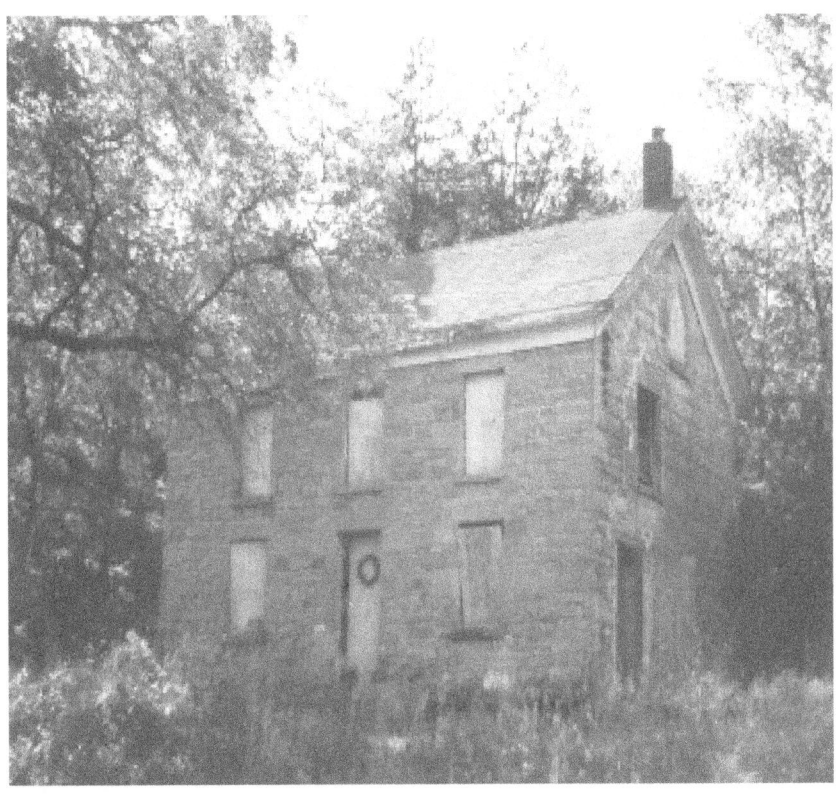

Home that Dennis Daniel McCarville built in 1863

Immigrants entering Wisconsin in Lafayette County signed a letter of intent. The document Dennis Michael McCarville signed in 1862 (incorrectly identifying him as junior) is housed in the Wisconsin Room University Archives of the Karrmann Library, University of Wisconsin- Platteville. " I, Dennis McCarville, Jr. do respectfully certify that I was born in the County of Monahan(*sic*) and within and in allegiance to Queen Victoria and am now 27 years of age; that I emigrated from Liverpool in said Kingdom and arrived at New York in the United States of America, in the month of December A.D. 1848; that I now reside in the county of Lafayette, in the State of Wisconsin, and it is bona fide my intention to become a citizen of the United States of North America, and to renounce all allegiance to every foreign King, Prince, Potentate and State and especially to Victoria Queen of Great Britain & Ireland.

State of Wisconsin,
LA FAYETTE COUNTY, ss.

I, Dennis McCarville, do respectfully certify that I was born in the County of Monahan, Ireland and within allegiance to Queen Victoria, and am now 27 years of age; that I emigrated from Liverpool in said Kingdom and arrived at New York in the United States of America, in the month of December A.D. 1848; that I now reside in the County of La Fayette, in the State of Wisconsin, and it is bona fide my intention to become a citizen of the United States of North America, and to renounce all allegiance to every foreign King, Prince, Potentate and State, and especially to Victoria Queen of Great Britian & Ireland.

Subscribed and sworn to before me, this 4th day of November A.D. 1862.

Dennis McCarville

Attest: James S. _____ Clerk
Circuit Court, La Fayette County, Wisconsin.

Dennis Michael McCarville was a citizen of the United States.

Chapter Three

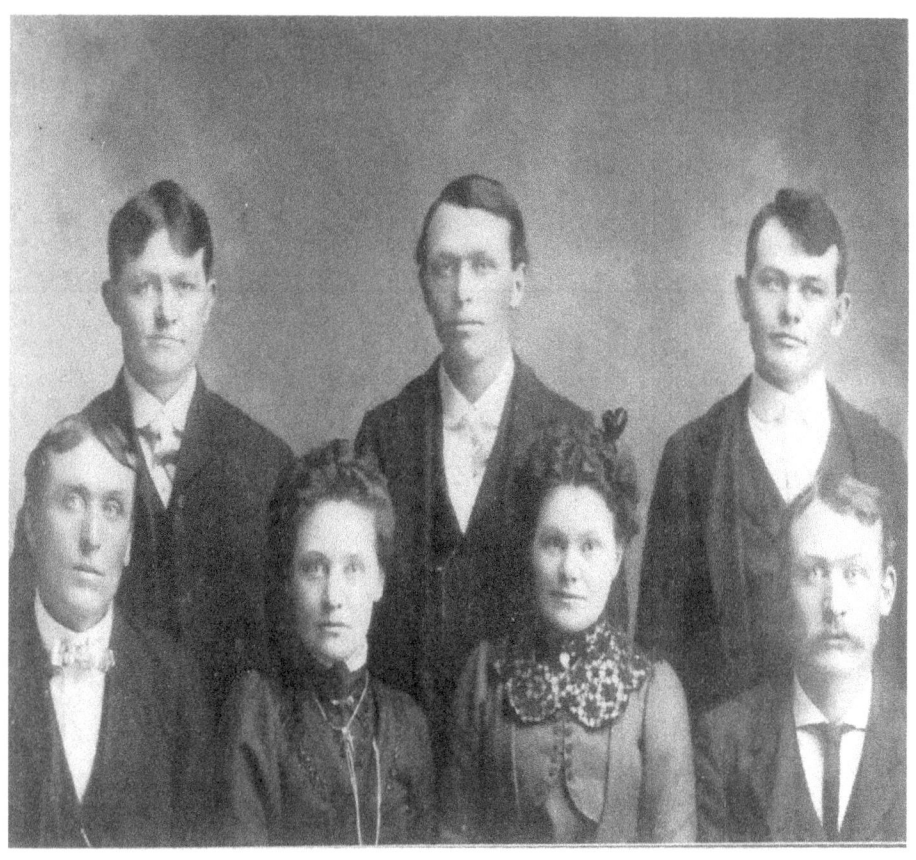

Children of Dennis Michael McCarville and Catherine Timmen 1900

Dominic, James, Joseph

Thomas, Mary Ann, Catherine, Dennis Luke

Dennis Michael and Catherine Timmen had seven children in Wisconsin and following Irish custom, named the first name of their third son after Dennis, a robust baby with brilliant blue eyes. Dennis Luke McCarville was born May 21 of 1868; this was Jack's grandfather. The seven children enjoyed the stone house in Wisconsin that grandfather Dennis Daniel had built.

During social events, people talked about a new law called the Homestead Act that allowed the sale of 160 acres in the west to any head of a household who was a citizen and agreed to cultivate the land for five years. Like other McCarville men before him, Dennis Michael was curious, inspired and motivated to change his future and that of his children. After mutual agreement with his sons and wife, he risked his entire finances on a homestead in Moorland, Iowa. Seven years after his father died, Dennis Michael sold his father's home and bought one section of 640 acres, paying $1.25 cash per acre, which was a large investment at the time.

Dennis Michael and Catherine thoroughly enjoyed an intense project of planning and building their own custom home in Moorland in 1890 on the northeast corner of the land. Following homestead requirements, the home was set back from the road with a long line of trees on both sides of the lane leading to the house. This farmland is now known as the "McCarville Section."

Tragically, the entire farmland was quickly divided up between the older four sons when Dennis Michael McCarville died suddenly on March 28, 1890 only a few weeks after moving to Moorland. He is buried at the Moorland Cemetery; his headstone indicating he died at the age of 55 years. The diagnosis of pneumonia is listed as his cause of death. Due to the medical care at the time of his death, the cause of pneumonia by the attending doctor would not be certain. Cultures, chest X-rays or blood tests such as white blood cell counts were not available. Infectious pneumonia often produces a high fever with shaking chills and colored sputum, which Dennis Michael suffered from before his death, but pneumonia can be viral, fungal or even chemical such as dust from cement. Doctors in Moorland at the time documented death on a mortality schedule, which contains various causes of death listed for the year to include "Dead Born", "Dropsy", "Bold Hives", "Flux" or "None". Pneumonia was a common cause of death before the advent of antibiotics as was diphtheria, measles, and tuberculosis.

Catherine was so devastated after her husband's death she never remarried. All the children lived in the original house in Moorland with Catherine until they married. However, her son James stayed and lived in the house with Catherine and his family when he married. Catherine died on May 5, 1918 at the age of 80 after helping to care for her children, many grandchildren and great grandchildren. Jack remembers playing around her headstone as a child in the Moorland cemetery.

When Dennis Luke was 22 years old, he married a beautiful dark haired Irish girl in 1895 named Mary Jane (Jennie) Halligan who was the daughter of Irish immigrants who were farmers in the area. Jennie's knew her grandfather Anthony I Halligan and grandmother Mary McKenna were from County Louth Ireland. Jennies father Anthony I Halligan, Jr. had married Anna Jennie and Dennis Luke in his late years. His Irish roots indicate his family came from Louth, Ireland which is He had nervously asked her to a dance after Mass in Moorland and met her numerous times at picnics, funerals and social activities. The town was happy to celebrate their marriage in January of 1895. Everyone in the area came and brought many wonderful gifts. The small town of Moorland was ready for the excitement of this young couple's wedding, which was a grand affair and talked about for many months after.

The marriage of Dennis McCarville and Jennie Halligan occurred at Moorland on Wednesday, January 9, 1895. After the ceremony the young couple with their friends were served to a bountiful wedding breakfast at the home of the bride's parents in Elkhorn township. Following is a list of the beautiful presents received. The MESSENGER unites with their friends in hearty congratulations.

Anthony Halligan - dining room set and bedroom set
James & Syd Halligan - cook stove
Mrs. D. McCarville, - rocking chair
Mollie McCarville - silver caster
Jas. McCarville - album
Domenic McCarville - cuff buttons and bedspread
D. Farrell and wife - set of dishes
Mrs. M. Savage - lamp
Lena Halligan - lamp
Jas. McCarville - toilet set
John McCarville - $1 cash
McCarville Bros. - table cloths
M. J. Welch & wife - hanging lamp
Wm Henzy and wife - glass water set
Joe McCarville - silver knives and forks
Will & Joe Mulroney - plush rocker
D. A. Halligan & wife - plush rocker
Jas Redden and wife - rocking chair
D. Crimmens - wash bowl and pitcher
Mrs. M. Crimmens - table cloth and napkins
S. J. Robertson - carving set
Maggie McCarville - mirror
M. Miller and wife - bedspread
D. J. Harrington - glass set
Frank McCarville - $1 cash
Will Blunck - flat irons
Alfred Loehr and wife - set silver spoons
T. A. McCarville and wife - set dining room chairs
Katie and Lizzie McCarville - lamp
Lizzie and Mary Dowling - plush rocker

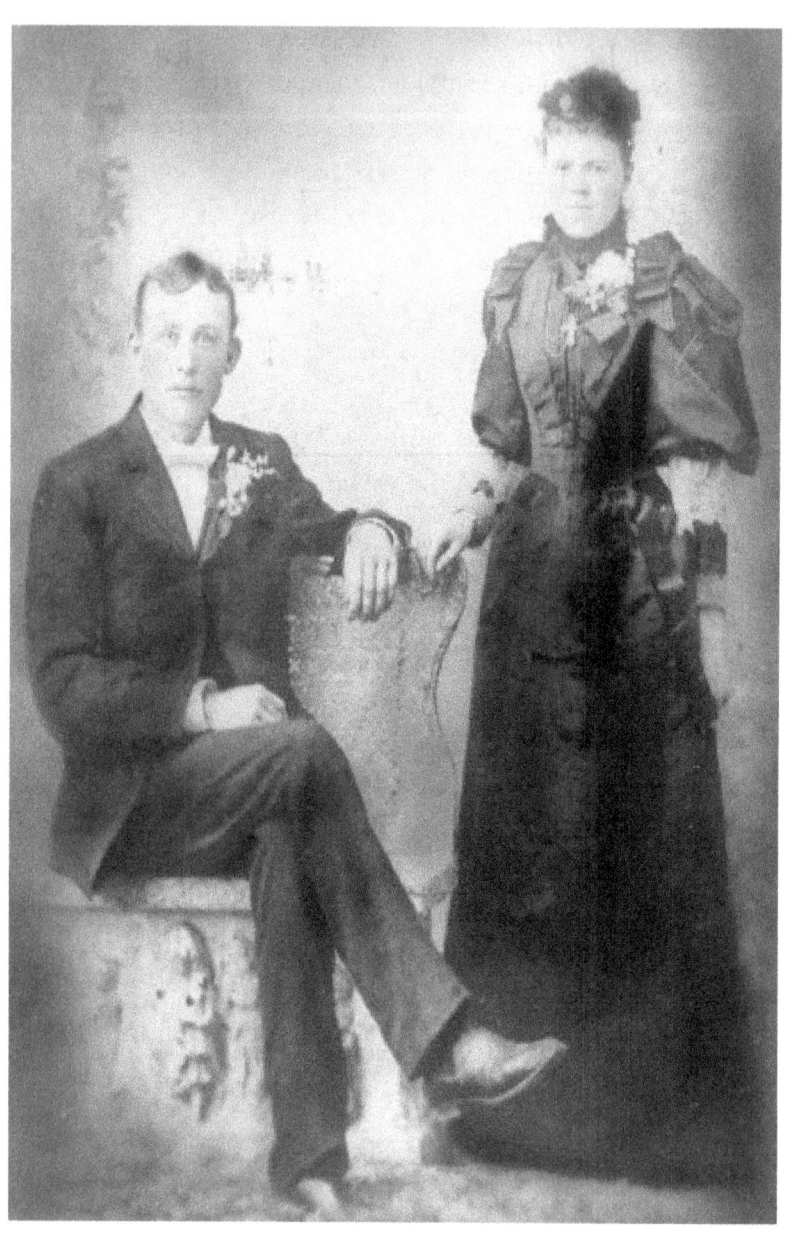

Dennis Luke McCarville and Mary Jane Halligan
Wedding Portrait
1895

No one at this time of joy could ever imagine the sorrow this couple would face in the future. Dennis Luke and Jennie had nine children. One was Jack's father Francis Joseph McCarville named after Saint Francis of Assisi, born October 20, 1901, a robust baby boy with brilliant blue eyes. Other children included Catherine, Eleanor, Genevieve, Anna, Cecelia, Robert, Raphael, and Anthony.

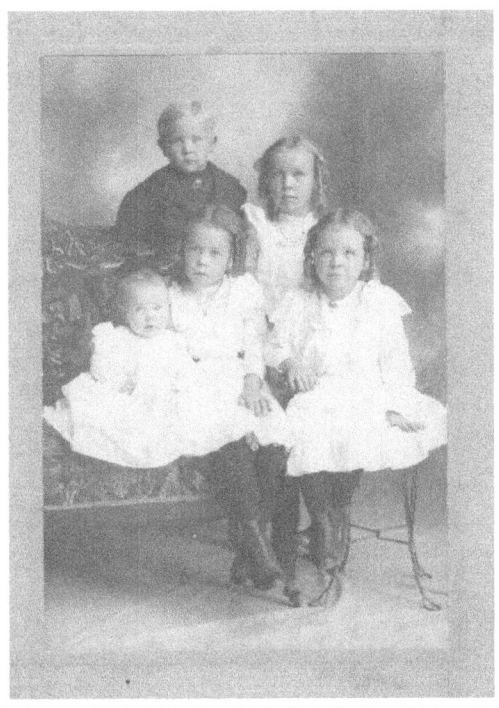

Children of Dennis Luke McCarville and Mary Jane Halligan
Francis, Mary Anne, Cecelia, Catherine, Genevieve
1904

Francis became close to his sister Catherine as they shared pain for the loss of their siblings in the family due to illness or disease. Catherine wrote Francis letters from her convent discussing the tragedy they experienced in their childhood together. She described how she remembered grieving for their small sister Mary Anne. She was unable to accompany her on their happy trek to school when she fell ill with appendicitis in late November of 1904 and remembers she "joined the angels" the next morning. She writes soon after that in 1905, when Catherine was at age six, she felt "desolate" when her younger sister Genevieve dies and "truthfully alone". Catherine writes in 1909 when she was ten and away at boarding school in Carroll, Iowa, a nun suddenly brought her into the office. She was told her five-year-old brother Anthony, "a chubby little fellow", had died. The cause of death was diphtheria, a contagious bacterial disease that causes a thick covering in the back of the throat. This disease can progress to breathing problems, heart failure, and death. Her sister Cecelia was seven and became ill at the same time as Anthony, and nearly died. Catherine remembers returning home after traveling alone in grief for a dreadful fifty miles from boarding school to find dear Anthony gone and her father by Cecelia's side in agony as she was hanging between life and death. Her entire body was shaking uncontrollably with tears streaming down her face as she prayed frantically outside the bedroom door when she heard her father shout out to God "I can surrender one child to my God if He will only spare the other!"

Miraculously, Cecelia lived. However, when she was 14 years old, she died from the terrifying "Spanish Flu" in the influenza pandemic of 1918. Her resistance against the flu was weak due to her previous battle with diphtheria. So many died from the pandemic flu that children on the street would skip rope to the rhyme "I had a little bird, its name was Enza, I opened the window and in-flu-enza". Funeral parlors soon found they could not keep up with the demand, as coffins were in short supply. Even President Woodrow Wilson battled the flu during the treaty of Versailles to end the First World War. People only went out in public with their faces covered with masks. The half million mortalities in the influenza pandemic were mostly young, healthy adults.

Each devastating funeral brought Catherine closer to her older brother Francis. The town watched them bravely console their parents bowed down with grief over the loss of each child. In between funerals, Catherine had the joy of receiving her First Holy Communion. In 1918, during the construction of Our Lady of Good Counsel Church in Moorland the community dedicated a stain glass window to Francis and his sister Catherine that still exists today. When Catherine attended high school at the St. Angela Academy in Carroll, Iowa, she made the decision to enter the religious life. Catherine would teach most of her life in the convent and her literary ability qualified her to judge children's books for publishers, which she enjoyed.

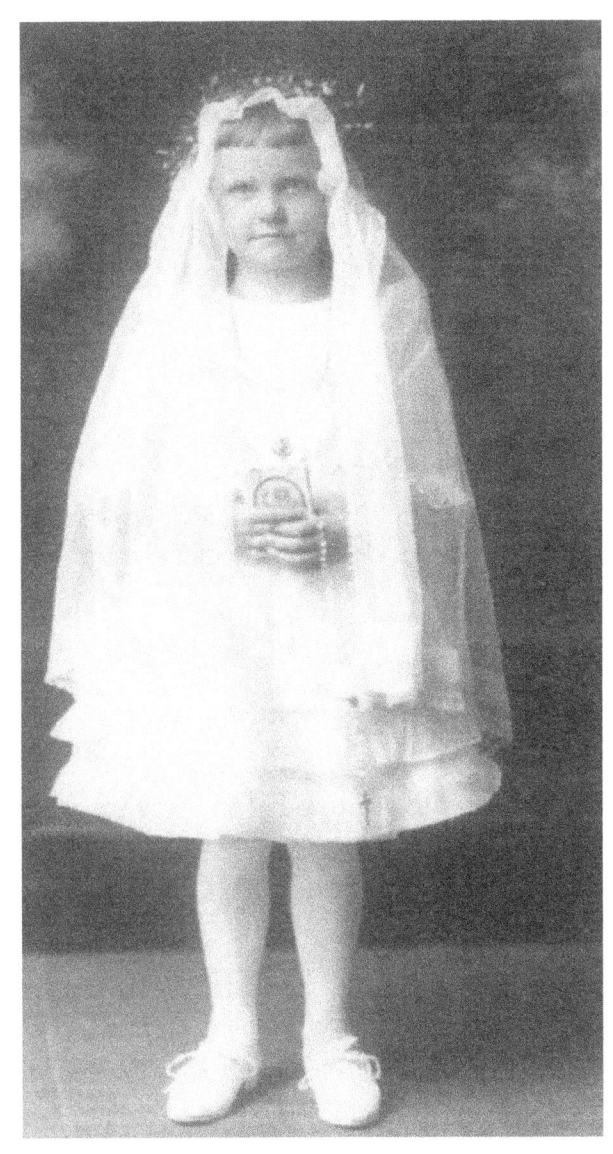

Catherine McCarville
First Holy Communion

Dennis Luke worked hard toward accomplishing his dream of providing a farm for each of his surviving sons, Francis, Robert and Raphael. In 1924, Francis was proud to be farming his own 180 acres across from the McCarville section, close in proximity to the home of his young cousin Ruth McCarville.

Francis had fallen in love with an Irish girl by the name of Catherine Bernice Coady born on February 25, 1902. He asked her to join him on a pheasant hunt and she agreed. She was so happy to spend time with the handsome Francis she never told him she absolutely hated guns until after they were married. Catherine was a third grade school teacher on the west side of town at the Moorland Consolidated School. She had graduated from Corpus Christi Roman Catholic High School in 1921.

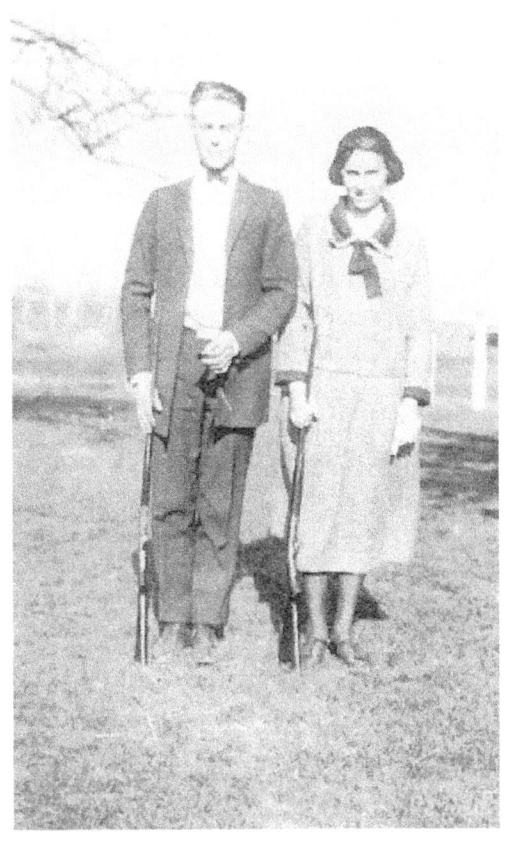

Francis McCarville and Catherine Coady
1923

One student of Catherine's was Ruth McCarville, the daughter of Joseph McCarville, one of the sons of Dennis Michael McCarville and Catherine Timmons. Known as Uncle Joe, he died from complications of diabetes at the age of 40 years due to the lack of insulin when Ruth was only four years old. Ruth lived on a farm on the southeast corner of the McCarville section and was upset when Catherine was going to marry, as the Moorland School District did not allow married women to teach. Ruth enjoyed Catherine as her third grade teacher and Catherine had to stop teaching in the middle of the year when she married.

The family tree of Catherine Bernice Coady includes her father John (also called Jack) Coady; he was born January 1, 1875. He came from a very large family of 16 children from Ivesdale, Illinois. His parents Patrick and Mary Walsh were from Ireland. Out of the 16 children they had, four of their sons died, three in infancy and one at the age of 21 due to the flu epidemic. All the other children lived to be elderly. Catherine's father Jack Coady married Catherine Hagen, a stunning Irish girl born May 10, 1876 who came from a well to do family in St. Louis.

Jack Coady and Catherine Hagen had five girls together: Mary, Catherine, Irene, Loretta and Josephine. These girls remember a very joyous childhood until tragedy struck the family when their mother gave birth to a stillborn baby boy in 1918. After the birth, the five girls watched in horror as their mother suffered for weeks before dying on July 15, 1918 from complications of pregnancy at the age of 42. Catherine was only 16 years old when her mother died and she was devastated, mourning for many years. Jack remembers his mother mourning this tragedy when he was a child.

Catherine hesitated when asked but acknowledged her father Jack Coady claimed the family name Coady was actually Cody originating from the family of William Frederick (Buffalo Bill) Cody born in 1846 in Iowa. Her father Jack was boisterous in his story of family members converting the spelling of Cody to Coady and the family relationship to Buffalo Bill. Years later, Catherine's grandson Patrick John McCarville at age 18 would bear a striking resemblance to

Buffalo Bill's military portrait at 19 years of age. Other famous relatives of Jack Coady indicate a relationship in the family tree to Button Gwinnett who signed the Declaration of Independence and the actor Gregory Peck.

Jack's parents, Catherine and Francis, married on February 20, 1924 in a beautiful church ceremony with a full Mass. Francis was proud to be providing Catherine with a two-story four bedroom wooden house that was moved from another location and placed over a previously built basement. Tradition brought family members together before a marriage, working until a home was ready for the new couple. Francis and Catherine stood on the porch of their beautiful new home and thanked everyone for their hard work. Although Catholic nuns were not allowed to leave the convent for family weddings at the time one picture was discovered that provides evidence of Sister Bernice attending her brother's wedding.

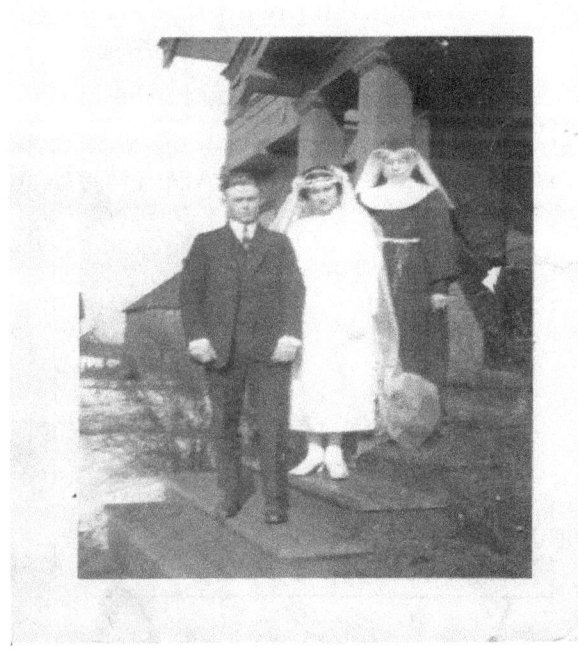

Francis and Catherine's wedding day in 1924 with Sister Bernice

Catherine missed her job as a teacher but was busy decorating her new house and helping Francis with the farm. She wrote letters to her family and enjoyed members of her husband's family as most lived near Moorland. Eight-year-old Ruth McCarville lived across the newly married couple's farm and would often visit her previous teacher Catherine. She remembers entertaining them by playing the piano and singing.

Ruth was excited to discuss her plans to attend Cedar Falls College and major in music. Everyone in the family had been proud when Ruth became part of the youngest orchestra in the State of Iowa in 1928.

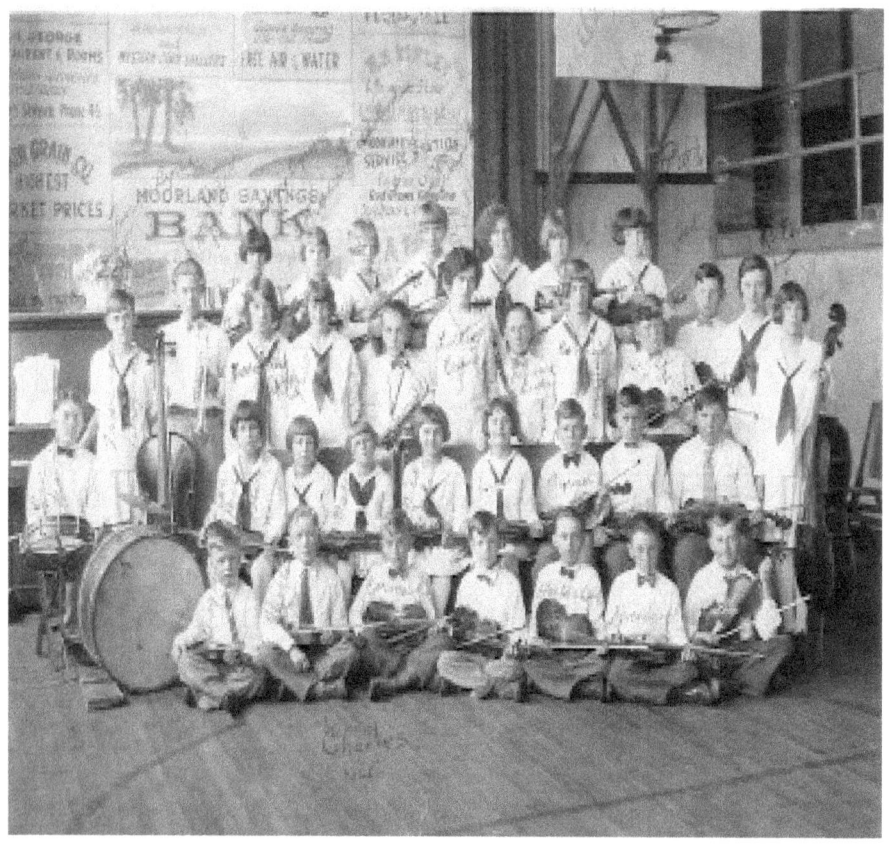

Ruth McCarville, Back Row, Last on the Right

1928

Dennis Luke had been able to accomplish his dream of his sons owning their own farms. Suddenly in 1929, the price for a bushel of corn fell to nine cents and farmers were in trouble as prices dropped over 60%. Instead of selling corn for profit, Dennis Luke used his corn for heating and cooking and his farm went into debt. Taxes rose, businesses closed in response to the taxation and unemployment was high.

Francis and his brother Robert were young and strong and assumed the responsibility of the debt of their father's farm during the Great Depression of the 1930's. When the Great Depression continued for years, young Ruth gave up her plans to go to college and have a career in music. She followed her sister Irene to the St. Rose Convent, to join the Franciscan Sisters who use the Rule of St. Francis of Assisi in their Motherhouse in the city of La Crosse, Wisconsin.

Francis was active in his spiritual life but worried about the reasons his sister Catherine and his cousin Ruth decided to enter the convent. He hoped it was not due to the fear of marriage and pain brought upon by the possible loss of those you love, such as a child, or a spouse. Although financial or marriage issues may have been a reason for women to seek the convent, Francis realized a special sense of freedom from stress the Sisters have that most people do not. Francis knew some people had a view that Catherine and Ruth suffered in some way, and they did not have a choice to leave once they entered the convent. They were very wrong.

When Ruth and Catherine entered the St. Rose Convent at the age of 18 years for their first year of postulancy, they did not wear a habit. They immediately began an education toward a college degree taught by other Sisters in the building. Ruth and Catherine began to practice teaching classes under the guidance of a Sister in a Catholic school across the street. A Sister who was a nurse cared for any medical problems and for other serious needs; St. Francis Hospital was just across the street.

Before the large Chapel of the Angels was built in 1906, individual wood and coal stoves in various places heated the Motherhouse. This could not be used in the large chapel so a boiler house had to be built which is still in use today. A tunnel was built for the hot water pipes to the Motherhouse and the hospital across the street. The tunnel was large enough for a person to walk through which was very helpful during the wintertime. The Sisters use the tunnel when it is snowing or raining to travel back and forth to the school or hospital. Today the Sisters have gone "green" as they use the steam plant to generate electricity in a process called combined heat and power. This method is more efficient and has less pollution. The Sisters grow their own fruits and vegetables in an organic garden.

Morning prayers were at five in the morning followed by Mass and then breakfast which was easily accomplished since farm girls were use to getting up early. Rosary was in the afternoon, after supper there was one hour of recreation before evening prayer, then everyone retired at nine in the evening. After one year Ruth and Catherine became novices, received a habit and veil and were given a Sister name. Ruth became Sister Virginia and Catherine became Sister Bernice. They were novices for two years, learning the three vows of poverty, chastity and obedience. They both worked at parish schools while completing their college degree. Many novices were interested in teaching or nursing and pursued degrees under the advice of the Superior; others were more comfortable with cooking or house work and became house Sisters, preparing meals and doing laundry. Summers allowed more time at the Motherhouse in the Chapel praying the Office in Latin in honor of the Blessed Virgin.

Sleeping quarters were in a dormitory with white cotton sheets separating individual sleeping areas for privacy. Each individual space for a Sister contained a bed, chair and a stand with a washbasin. The stand held clothing at the bottom and at the top was the basin for washing. Bathrooms were down the hall and each Sister was assigned a twenty-minute time once a week for a full bath. Every night the Sister filled her basin with water from the bathroom to take to their individual area. Years later, nuns were allowed individual rooms with shared bathrooms and upon retirement were allowed to choose their own private room with a bathroom.

Although Catherine was older than Ruth, both entered the convent at 18 years of age and were allowed to visit their family every five years; there were no exceptions for weddings or funerals. However, family members could visit at any time and they could choose to leave the convent forever without restriction. After two years as novices, renewal vows were made every three years and still, the Sisters could leave at any time, but very few Sisters left. Six years after entering the convent, final vows are made. If a Sister wishes to leave after final vows, she can but must obtain permission from Rome. Very few ever left the convent.

Francis went to visit his sister at her convent after his first child; Robert Francis McCarville was born in 1924. He was excited to bring her a picture of the baby. His previous life experiences in Iowa and Omaha did not prepare him for his travel to La Crosse, Wisconsin. He was amazed at the lush green trees and rolling hills, the Mississippi River and the incredible beauty of the city of La Crosse. He arrived on a Saturday by train and rested in his room on Main Street, getting up early to walk to the Saint Rose Convent to join the Sisters for Mass. A group of fifty Sisters including Sister Bernice and two cousins, Sister Patrice and Sister Agnelia met Francis in the lobby. After hugs of joy, they formed a line to walk into the chapel for Mass. As Francis walked behind the Sisters, they began to sing before they filed into the chapel. He walked slowly and looked up to his left as he passed an incredible statue of Saint Michael at the entrance to the chapel. As Francis followed their procession into the Chapel of the Angels, he felt as if angels were singing from above; their voices were so beautiful. Then he gasped. Nothing prepared him for the artistic and architectural beauty of what he was looking at when he first entered inside. High ceilings with over 100 windows of Bavarian stained glass are included in the Romanesque style of the Chapel of the Angels with many bronze statues. Huge Corinthian pillars are beside the main altar made of gold bronze, pillars of onyx, Italian marble with inlaid mosaics of mother of pearl and Venetian glass. Large rose patterns of circular stained glass window skylights portray the Holy Spirit of God surrounded by the heads of winged cherubs. Each pew is hand carved, made of red oak with a symbol of Mary, a rose and Greek cross. A virtual flash tour of what Francis experienced when he entered the chapel is on http://www.fspa.org/Prayer/maryofangelschapel/index.html

Sister Virginia admits the Sisters have a belief of a possible miracle of Saint Michael protecting the chapels from fire. One year a huge fire burned down the convent but stopped at the statue of Saint Michael, the chapels were spared. Stories come from others who insist the Sisters made a difference in the health of a loved one after the Sisters have prayed for them. Jack made a trip in 2008 to visit the grave of his Aunt Sister Bernice and meet with Sister Virginia at La Crosse, Wisconsin. After attending Mass in the Chapel of the Angels he was blessed to "go with angels" by Sister Virginia and Sister Rosalio Bauer of FSPA. Sister Virginia in the pictures below in June of 2008 shows Jack how to play the harp, the national emblem of Ireland.

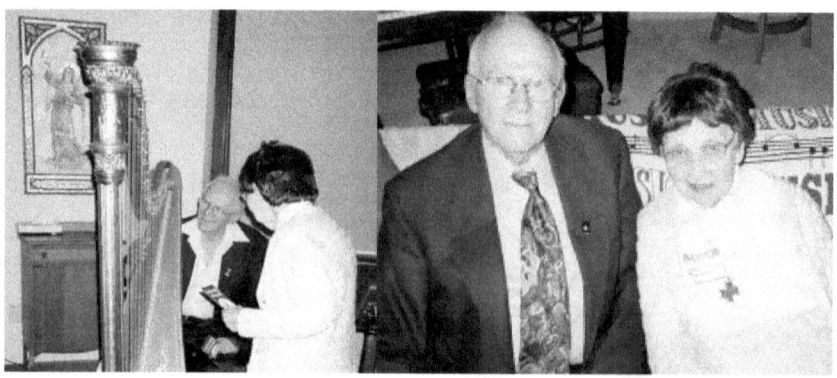

The Sisters live very long, happy and productive lives. When Sister Bernice or Sister Virginia did return home every five years, they would visit Catherine, Francis, and their growing family. Ruth (Sister Virginia) resides today in La Crosse, Wisconsin at the St. Rose Convent and has recently celebrated her 70th Jubilee. Four cousins who became nuns, originally from Moorland, Iowa lived at the St Rose Convent in Lacrosse, Wisconsin at the same time.

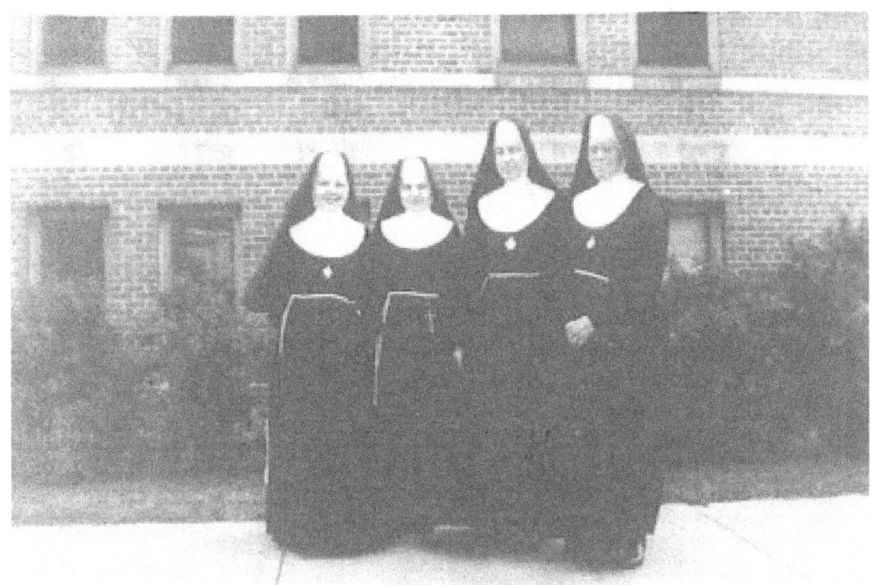

Sister Agnelia (Gertrude) McCarville, Sister Virginia (Ruth) McCarville, Sister Patrice (Lucille) Halligan and Sister Bernice (Catherine) McCarville.

The gravesite of "Father Joe" a grandson of Dennis Daniel McCarville, who became a priest, is in Clare, Iowa a small town near Moorland where Jack's wife Margaret Yetmar was born. Immigrants from Clare County Ireland settled Clare, Iowa around 1882. Joseph Hyginus McCarville studied for the priesthood at Creighton University in Omaha and said his first Mass in Clare at Saint Matthews Catholic Church. Tradition holds a priest to be buried where he says his first Mass. Father Joseph traveled to Ireland on many occasions spending numerous hours searching all parish records in County Monaghan for information on the McCarville family. He collected data interviewing the town's people and drew accurate and extensive family trees. He found all McCarville clans centered on Greenan Cross, a country crossroads a few miles from the town of Monaghan. Ireland has four provinces that are divided into thirty-two counties. The McCarvilles lived in Monaghan County in the Province of Ulster. Ireland, known as the Emerald Isle, at any location on the island is less than

100 miles from the sea. The information Father Joe was able to obtain in Ireland was important for the McCarville family tree. During the years of English rule, census recordings of the Irish were not performed as the Irish were regarded as "non-persons". Father Joe died at the young age of 48 years from tuberculosis.

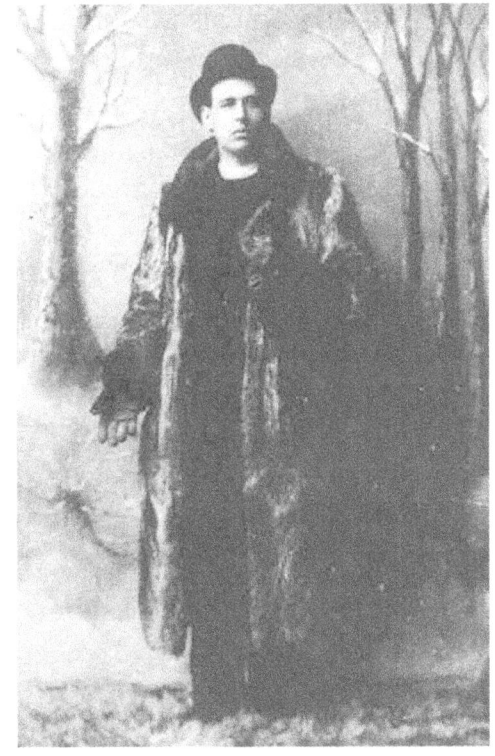

Father Joseph H. McCarville

When Francis and Catherine married, they were fortunate to have a home modern for that time. A hot oil stove in the living room kept the upper levels of the home warm as the heat drifted up through registers on the second floor. A wooden stove in the kitchen kept five gallons of water hot in a reservoir to provide basin baths for the family using handmade soap from ingredients of lye and lard. Twice a year Catherine made soap by collecting drippings from hog fat from pan-frying and heating it in a large black iron kettle outside over a fire. She added lye to the lard and mixed the liquids together until thick, pouring the mixture into heavy cardboard boxes. After cooling, Catherine cut the slabs into thick heavy bars. The bars had to cure for a week before using. Catherine had a total of 13 pregnancies, but only 8 living children. Whether a miscarriage or live birth, each of the 13 times she was pregnant she spent 10 days at Mercy Hospital in Fort Dodge with the exception of three children Bernard, Bud and Steven, who had been born at home. Jack, Tommy, Mary

Catherine, Danny, and Francis Anne were born at the hospital. Catherine was 43 years old when her last child Francis Anne was born.

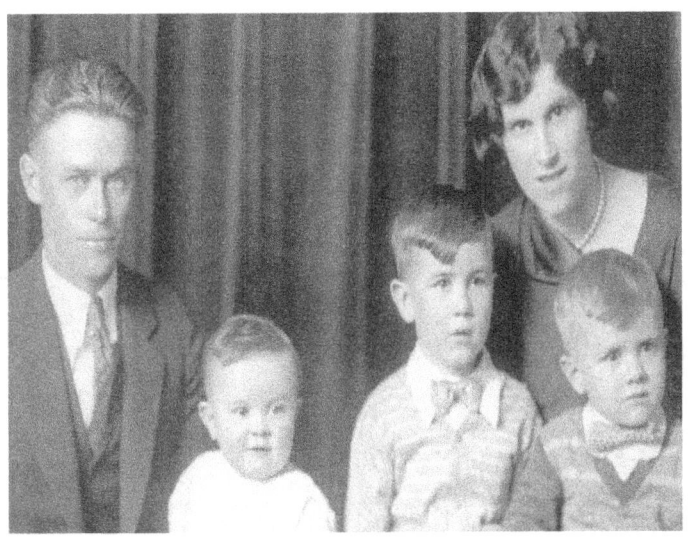

Francis, Bernard, Robert, Catherine and Jack McCarville
1929

Mercy Hospital was located in Fort Dodge, Iowa, operated by a religious order of Catholic nuns from their Motherhouse in Detroit, who wore the traditional black robes of the order, the Sisters of Mercy. These nuns were "walking nuns" as they lived outside the walls of a convent and worked with the public. The order was established in Ireland in 1831, founded by Mother Catherine McCauley with a sacred mission to provide health care to immigrants throughout the world and introduce the Catholic faith. Hospitals at this time were often operated by a religious organization and financial funding came from charitable donations or public funds. Staffing was made up of healthcare workers who were willing to work for less than prevailing market salaries as the emphasis was on providing healthcare for the indigent sick.

The year of 1936 was a difficult year for the McCarville family as they weathered an unusual cold spell. Joseph Halligan, the 36-year cousin of Francis, who was the best man at his wedding, died from a heart attack in Roelyn while shoveling snow as he was attempting to deliver mail. Francis found funerals difficult to attend especially after his siblings died from a combination of appendicitis, diphtheria and influenza. These painful memories prompted Francis to be proactive in the health needs of his family. He worked hard to pay for the services of the family doctor Thomas Dorsey from the nearby city of Fort Dodge. Francis never failed to pay the doctors or the hospital for their charges but knew they would never turn anyone away, regardless of their ability to pay. Before calling the doctor from Fort Dodge to come out to the house for help, Catherine and Francis would try the current home remedies for various ailments. This could be chicken soup, cod liver oil, rubbing alcohol, vinegar or aspirin. If necessary, a trip into town to consult with the pharmacist could solve the problem, such as an eye drop for an eye infection.

Jack knew early on he wanted to be a doctor but not because of any particular person in his life. He just knew that was what he wanted to do. Jack had his tonsils out by Dorsey and would often be examined by him for his wheezing which he had ever since he was sick at the age of two with bacteria called Pertussis commonly known as "whooping cough." This disease causes violent coughing spells, rib fractures and weight loss but Jack had been a robust and strong boy before he became ill. He was able to survive, while most children who had this disease did not. Pertussis could easily progress to pneumonia and death. Francis was vigilant and never left Jack's bedside while he ill. Jack survived but had problems with episodes of severe wheezing. Catherine took trips into Fort Dodge with Jack to discuss this problem with the doctor. Dr. Dorsey smoked a cigarette in the examination room as he explained Jack's current condition, called asthma. Jack observed Dorsey with great interest and heard him talking with his mother about a disease that his father's Uncle Joe had died from, called diabetes.

Jack knew his father's cousin Ruth McCarville as she lived across their farm before she left for the convent. Ruth was only four years old when her father died but she does have one memory of him sitting in a large rocking chair by the bay window. She remembers his casket in the living room but she did not understand the concept of death. Uncle Joe believed in educating his children and sent his son to Creighton Prep in Omaha and Ruth's older sister Irene to a domestic science school taught by the Franciscan Sisters of Perpetual Adoration in La Crosse, Wisconsin. Sister Bernice taught Irene and escorted her home from school each summer. The rules of the convent were strict about family visits but Sister Bernice took every opportunity available to visit her brother and his growing family. Even as a child, Jack knew how important his Aunt Sister Bernice was to his father.

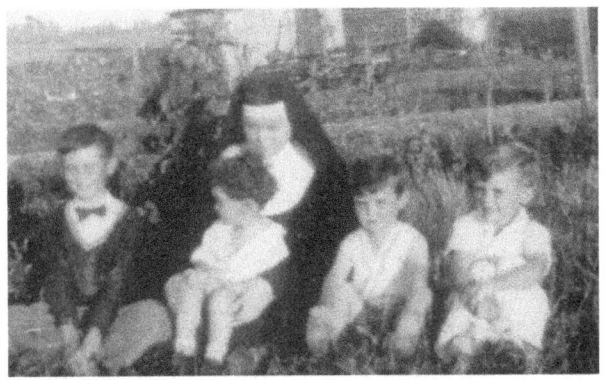

Robert (Bud), Sister Bernice, Steve, Bernard and Jack
1933

Doctor Dorsey diagnosed Ruth's father Joe with diabetes after he had lost weight and was urinating more than normal. He would drink large quantities of liquid but was unable to quench his thirst. Dr. Dorsey used the term polyuria for the frequent urination and polyphagia for his uncontrollable urges to eat. If Joe did eat pie or cake he became dizzy, tired and would complain of nausea and blurry vision. Dr. Dorsey explained the sugar was so thick in his body that the fluid was pulling on the lens in his eyes and distorting his vision. Insulin did not exist yet and Joe died at the young age of 40 years from the disease. Joe's son Eugene developed Type I diabetes, but he survived as insulin was developed during his lifetime.

Jack remembers being in the kitchen cutting a cake he had made for the family and was amused as he watched his father Francis counsel the family dog a Saint Bernard named Barney who was muddy and on the front landing of the house trying to gain entrance. Jack watched Barney's birth as a puppy and years later kept him warm in the basement when he died. There were 40 cats on the farm to keep the mice population down and occasionally a mouse would scamper across the bedclothes in the dark of night. During the cold winter months, Francis occasionally brought in hatchlings, a piglet or a lamb to keep warm next to the oil stove. Francis sent the wool from his sheep away for cleaning to make quilts for the beds during the winter.

Francis had six large Belgium horses that pulled equipment, as he did not have a tractor. In the famously cold winter of 1936, he used his horses to pull a snow sled to help him do the work of the farm. Francis woke up very early in the morning and did most of the work himself. He was relieved to have his oldest son Bud help him with the heavy farm work when he was older as the other boys did when they came of age, except for Jack.

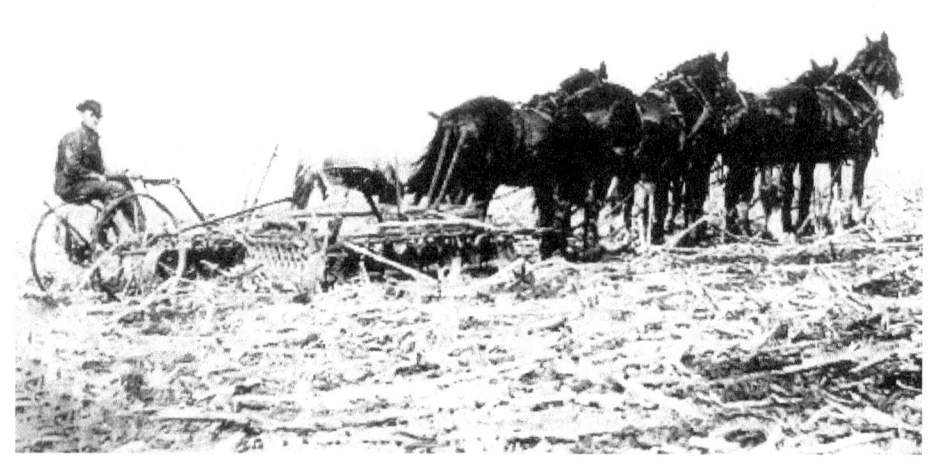

Francis working on the farm
1936

The best part of the day for Francis was dinner with his family as the very hard work of the farm was over for the day, and he could relax. Many times the children grabbed the bat, baseball mitt and ball and played a game. Francis taught Bernard and Steve to box and they soon started to compete in the boxing ring in town. Francis and Catherine enjoyed listening to entertainment programs on an Atwater Kent radio. Jack remembers some programs were similar to soap operas. The radio had three batteries and vacuum tubes. Francis loved to play cards and became an expert in the game of bridge.

Francis grew and sold corn for 10 cents a bushel, oats as a cash crop and alfalfa hay for his horses. Francis was careful to improve and keep the superior quality of his corn crop. Every year in the fall, he would pick out the best ears of corn and test for seed quality for the next year. He shelled the ears and planted them in a test tray to see how strong the seed was before bagging the targeted ears for seed for the next year. As corn ripens in the fields, the wind swirls the pollen and cross-pollinates. The neighbors of Francis who grew corn benefited from the high quality of his corn from this cross-pollination process.

Francis sold calves of high quality and sought to achieve an even higher grade of stock with the introduction of new blood in his herds each year. He raised and sold pigs and shot a few pigs for the family to eat in the freezing weather, as the meat would keep as long as it stayed cold. Jack asked his father if he could shoot the pig chosen for the family and Francis took extra time to show him the exact target area. Jack missed his head and shot him in the neck instead, which made the pig mad and Francis mad. Jack would not find out he needed glasses for his distant vision until he was 17 years old. Pigs provided the family bacon and hams, which they cured with a dry salt rubbed on the meat multiple times for several weeks. The intestines were used for sausage casing, which was fried and placed in large crocks and covered with lard. Leftover scraps of meat were ground up, mixed with barley and mashed potatoes and pressed down solid in a crock for frying for breakfast. No part of the meat was wasted.

The family had over 80 leghorn chickens in a large chicken house within walking distance of the house to use for family meals. Leghorn chickens are noisy and capable of flying but are known for their positive egg production. Excess eggs were traded for supplies at the store in town. The children knew not to kill the large bull snakes that curled up and slept in the nests of the chicken house as they devoured rats and the never-ending supply of mice around the corn barn. The chickens did not lay eggs as much in the winter; therefore, in the fall, Catherine would fill three 20-gallon crocks with strong salt water and carefully place fresh eggs in the crock to have enough to eat through the winter. There was a beautiful garden near the house the children and Catherine tended. In the summer, Catherine would can a colorful collection of a vast variety of fruits and vegetables and store a huge supply in the basement that would last all winter.

Francis would often sit on the porch on the front of the house after dinner. If a neighbor passed by, they would wave to each other. Catherine's father Jack Coady would sit on the porch with Francis during his visits to the family. He would use his cane to grab a grandchild around the neck as they passed by. When he pulled them forward toward him, he would give them a piece of candy corn. There was no crime in the area but on occasion transients would boldly enter the property and steal chickens and eggs. Neighbors would help each other when needed and sometimes there were accidents on the farms. Horses would bolt and some of the farming equipment was dangerous to use. Candles or kerosene lamps were used for light that was flammable.

When the children were small, the younger children took their bath two at a time in a big metal washbasin by the stove. Outhouses on farms were set in the back of the house over a hole dug in the ground of about six feet down. When the hole filled up, Francis covered the area over with dirt and moved the outhouse over to a freshly dug hole. During cold winter nights, the family used pots in the house to relieve themselves; which had to be emptied in the outhouse in the morning. Occasionally, the younger boys would accidently spill their pots on the way with evidence seen as a colorful trail in the snow the next day.

Frances had a separate fruit grove with mulberry bushes, apple and cherry trees planted near the side of the house. A large barn for the horses was near another barn for corn. There was an old barn still standing before the other buildings were built now used to store hay. Several large trees planted close to the house to fulfill homestead requirements provided shade and wind protection. Jack learned how to cook while helping his mother in the kitchen when he had to stay home from school and became quite a chef. Catherine spent a great deal of time with Jack and he learned most of her recipes; his favorite was her one-egg cake and homemade fudge on the stove. He checked the temperature of the fudge with a mercury thermometer to make sure it was just right temperature before he took it off to cool. Jack cooked a breakfast of bacon, eggs, potatoes and hot bread topped with fresh butter every Saturday for the family and cleaned up afterward. Jack cooked fresh eggs just gathered from the chicken house with the yellow yolks standing up high in grease from the bacon he cooked first. All the bacon grease went into a thick blue Mason jar kept by the stove to be used later for making soap. During the week, everyone was in a hurry and did not have time for a full breakfast so a bowl of hot fresh bread pieces, hot oatmeal, or cooked white rice pudding with raisins, sugar and fresh milk was prepared.

Francis had eight milk cows and brought Jack pails of milk from the cows early in the morning to pour into a separator on the porch that was a big bowl, attached to a funnel leading to a machine turned by a crank. Jack turned the crank and a centrifuge separated the cream from the skim milk; he transferred this cream into a glass churn with wooden paddles that turned to make a light colored butter. It took about 30 minutes of turning the paddles before Jack heard the thump indicating butter had formed. Any remaining liquid was buttermilk; Jack drained this off to make cottage cheese. He did this by setting a bowl of the churned buttermilk into the icebox on the porch for few days. Francis would buy a large block of ice from town or sometimes use ice he found in the nearby creek to keep the tin lined box cold. During the depression, many people in the city would go hungry but life on the farm had the advantage of a good supply of food.

After he finished his chores with the milk, Jack spent most of the day reading in his bedroom if he was wheezing and avoided the outdoors. Blowing dust would cause a constriction in his throat and he annoyed others with his persistent cough and wheezing. He vomited when it became too much of a struggle and his mother put him in a warm bath with menthol until he calmed down. The vapors of steam from the bath seemed to help; afterwards he went to his room where he felt safe. He did not cough as much in his room that Catherine kept very clean. Sometimes his mother lit a green powder and the smoke would help him cough up his congestion. He often used a device with a glass tube called a nebula that used a rubber bulb to administer a medication to open up his lungs.

Strangely, Jack found he could jump up on his Shetland pony Tony and ride without coughing much. However, when he went into the stalls and barn, he immediately started wheezing. To ride Tony he grabbed the thick black hair on his mane, slung his long skinny leg over and sharply kicked the left side and suddenly, he became one with the horse. He rode bareback and one time proudly took fifth in a race at church even after being bucked off at the starting lineup. Jack had no concept of fear when he rode in a race or through the roads next to the cornfields that seemed to go on forever. He was free to ride as fast as he could with nothing to stop him and neighbors smiled when they saw the duo flying by. Jack was slight but tall and felt an immense power and control while riding that was exhilarating to him. Being in his room so much gave him an urgent sense of adventure whenever he was able to be out of the house.

Jack's childhood social life around the farm included playing with the neighbor boy Jimmy Ferrin who was being raised by his grandmother. The usual sport for the family was baseball and his brothers were excellent boxers. Jack had a cousin Paul, who was his own age and slept at the house for a few days. They enjoyed playing war games. They used pillowcases as parachutes to jump off the porch, flung fruit as ammunition and used oatmeal boxes to bang on as drums. Many times, they ran through the clothes Catherine was hanging up with wooden pins to dry in the outside air that had taken hours for her to wash. Catherine had three or four heavy flat irons kept hot on the wood stove for ironing. If they became hungry, they grabbed an apple off the tree or a tomato from the garden. Carrots, raw potatoes and watermelon were favorites of Jack's and he sprinkled salt on everything. Once, they went to a nearby creek to fish and Catherine saved the fish for Friday. Catherine made two full meals a day for Francis, one at noon and one at supper with meat, potatoes, vegetables and fresh bread provided at each meal. She made cakes and pies on Saturdays - all from scratch. A favorite dessert in Moorland was her poppy seed cake with soft butter on the side. Catherine was a diligent housekeeper and even more devout Catholic. Everything seemed to revolve around their Catholic faith and Jack respected every part of the family routine of daily prayer, rosary and the trips into town for church.

Every Sunday before Mass, one of the children had an unsavory chore to accomplish in the chicken house. The children had to take turns catching a young plump chicken to prepare for dinner. The chickens ate ground corn but were allowed to roam and kept healthy chasing the bugs and eating the grass. Chopping off a chicken's head required skill with the axe and getting out of the way quickly as the chicken hopped for a while even after the head was gone. Rather than the axe, the younger children would ring the chicken's neck then pull the feathers off in a messy stack before bringing it to

Catherine. She then dipped the chicken in boiling water to remove the rest of the pinfeathers. Catherine baked a chicken dinner every Sunday and the family looked forward to this after Mass as they fasted before Communion and were hungry.

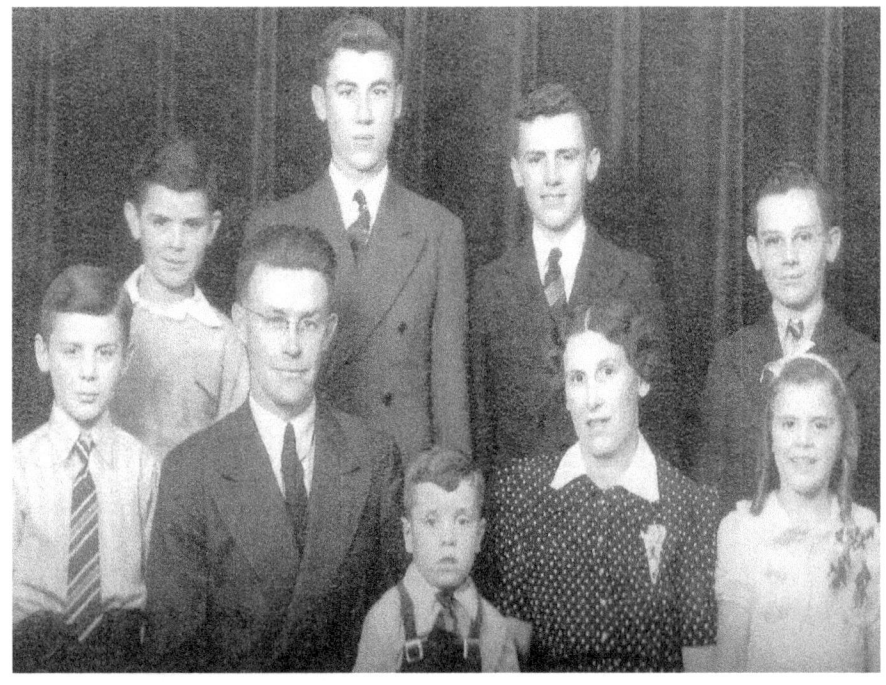

Front: Thomas, Francis, Daniel, Catherine, Mary Catherine
Back: Steven, Robert, John (Jack) and Bernard
1941

Sometimes Jack felt he was a prisoner in his own bedroom due to his asthma. Jack realized the books he was reading did not match the life he was living on the farm. His books were a portal to a world no one in his family knew existed. He was learning to play the accordion during the day as he had gone to the Bohemian Hall in Fort Dodge and seen a musician he was very impressed with, a man named Lawrence Welk. He was able to attend school about one fourth of the time at the Moorland Consolidated School on the west side of town. The school had bus service and playground equipment. Most of the students who attended the school were children of farmers with different backgrounds. The children from the west of Moorland were Norwegian, the Bohemians lived southeast and the German and Irish lived in the middle areas. When Jack was unable to attend school, a teacher named Miss Kline provided Jack with books from class. She would send them home with Jack's siblings; he would finish one book and send it back only to wait for another. Miss Kline was amazed at the amount and type of books Jack was able to read so quickly and discussed this with Francis and Catherine. He could read a book she would be teaching all semester to her students in 10 days. When she would quiz him on the book, he was correct on any question. When she ran out of books in his age group, she gave him other books she thought he would enjoy. He marveled at science and biology and was amazed at the microscope he observed in Dr. Dorsey's office.

Father Bernard Hunt, an Irish priest from County Cork in the Province of Munster, Ireland said Mass at Our Lady of Good Counsel in Latin with the use of incense. Father Hunt had a large library and served the Church for 32 years. After Mass while chatting with the parishioners, he would say how he missed Ireland, the green rolling hills, daily rain and rainbows. Jack learned from Father Hunt that Saint Patrick was responsible for the Irish converting to Christianity and was considered the most important man in Ireland who ever lived. St. Patrick used the shamrock to explain the concept of Trinity, the Father, Son and the Holy Ghost to the Irish.

Francis was a member of the Knights of Columbus to the Fourth Degree, an organization of Catholic men founded by Father Michael J. McGivney. This organization promotes social interaction, charity projects and spreads the faith of the Catholic Church. Francis enjoyed the social functions and working in the various projects to help the sick, elderly, poor, orphans and widows. Jack loved the uniform his father wore which was a tuxedo with white shirt and gloves, bow tie and an amazing black navy type chapeau with a colorful white plume. Best of all, Jack loved the silver sword his father wore at the side of this uniform. When Francis died, Jack asked for his father's Knights of Columbus uniform and has kept it to this day. Jack became a Fourth Degree Knights of Columbus member himself in Arizona.

Before Jack graduated from the Moorland Consolidated High School with a class of 17, he had taken a national high school test given by the navy who drafted students who did well on the exam to work on the submarines fighting the Germans in the North Pacific. During World War II, essential occupations such as farming were exempted from the draft but Francis felt this was unpatriotic and wanted all his sons to serve. Although all of his boys would serve in the U.S. Army, Bud was the only son to face combat. The rest of the boys Francis had said were "ground pounders". The U.S. Navy selected Jack as their draft as he had one of the highest scores ever. A crew of uniformed officers scheduled a meeting at the farm to interview him. They were surprised at his slight build next to the other hefty sons of Francis and found he could not pass a physical. This was a big embarrassment for Jack as his family had given him a going away party before he flunked the physical. Looking back now, it probably saved his life.

Chapter Four

Catherine and Francis decided it was best for Jack's health to send him to Arizona State Teachers College, now known as Arizona State University (ASU), in Tempe, Arizona. Jack applied for prerequisite classes for his desired medical degree in chemistry, physics, anatomy and sociology. In addition, he was required to take German in case he became physically eligible for the draft, due to the war. Jack left with one of Catherine's cakes in a box tied with a string, and one hundred dollars in cash, which was a great deal of money at the time. He never looked back. Jack realized on his first trip out of Iowa on a Greyhound bus to a place called Arizona, he had a unique happiness to travel. He found he was curious and willing to take risks. He did not miss his family; he was on an expedition and could not wait until the next adventure in his life came around the corner.

Jack rode the bus for hours looking out the window at all the sights he was driving by; he could not sleep in case he would miss something. When it became dark, he dozed off and the bus reached Tempe late in the night. He had been amazed at the sights of strange looking palm trees, purple colored mountains and cacti called Saguaro. Although it was late in the evening, he was shocked at the blast of dry heat similar to an oven as he stepped off the bus. He soon realized this dry heat would be much more comfortable for him to breathe in than the humidity of a summer in Iowa. He was thankful to realize a man from the college was waiting for him at the bus station to drive him to his dormitory. After a short trip, he was introduced to a situation very new in his life but one he would become used to for many years- a dormitory roommate. His first roommate was Joe Espinoza, whose mother's name was Mason, a young man from a prestigious family in Hermosillo, Mexico.

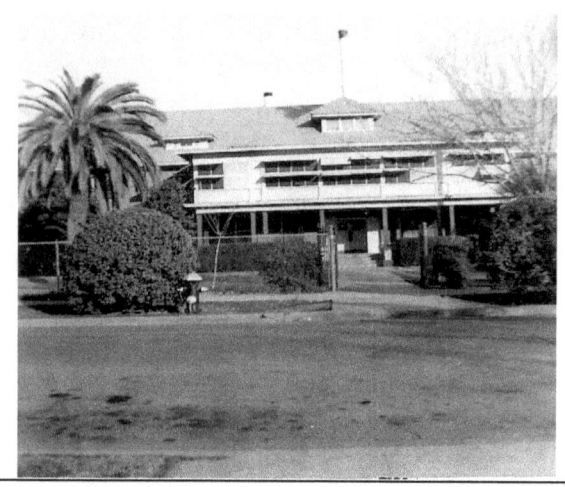

College Dormitory in Tempe, Arizona where Jack stayed in 1945

Jack signed in for his classes, toured the campus and settled into his new routine of school in a college dormitory in a very different place. Jack was happy with his new life but suddenly struggled with insomnia. He began a daily ritual of exercise climbing mountains. This he would do until much later in his life. He began to climb a mountain near the college now known as "A" mountain in the late afternoon. At the end of his climb as he reached the top of the mountain, he would sit on a flat rock and marvel at the colorful pink and blue sunsets. Sometimes the sun would appear red against a sky with so many colors he could not describe the beauty to his family. After only a few months, Jack was determined to make his home in Arizona. He enjoyed the unique beauty and wildlife of the desert especially the birds such as the roadrunner, which looked to Jack like a desert chicken. Quails ran in single file groups with strange colorful plumes on their heads, always protecting their family. Wild rabbits were everywhere peeking up out of holes and running about. Jack saw desert tortoises; lizards called geckos and horny toads, which had the appearance of wearing armor, but were easy to catch. Although warned, Jack never encountered a rattlesnake until years later when his son Thomas was bitten after picking up a baby rattlesnake when the family was at an outing at Lake Pleasant. Jack wrapped his young son's hand in a cold towel and prayed the long hour it took to drive him to the nearest hospital where his treatment was successful.

Jack saw many skinny wild dogs called coyotes; but some were heavier with thick coats and looked like wolves.

They woke him up late in the night with loud yelps and strange cries as they ran in groups catching rabbits. One morning on the way to class, he saw a bobcat mother with her baby struggling behind her while dragging a small rabbit in its mouth. One early evening a huge owl with a face the size of a dinner plate swooped suddenly out of a crevice in the mountain Jack was climbing, he turned and marveled at the wingspan as he flew away. Jack was amazed at the different species of cactus; some have large exotic white flowers that only bloom at night. Birds were also different in Arizona- mockingbirds kept everyone awake many nights. Jack thought they must be playing cards when they chanted "shuffle, shuffle, shuffle, deal, deal, deal" next to his window at two in the morning.

    Jack would not return home until the next summer and wrote often about his experiences to his family and friends. He had an intense postal relationship with his Aunt Sister Bernice who encouraged him on in his studies. He looked forward to her letters, as she never failed to write words of support and later on in his life, he would remember her as giving him unconditional love. She was a sensitive, intelligent teacher and they would exchange discussions and ideas about the world. She truly cared about Jack and they continued to write to each other on a regular basis for many years until shortly before she died in 1966. Jack wrote that the countryside and rainy weather of Ireland must be the exact opposite of where he was living in Arizona. She agreed that he was living in weather completely different from where her grandfather was from and there were no snakes in Ireland. Jack's children grew up with a picture of Aunt Sister Bernice in their house and he would share her letters with them.

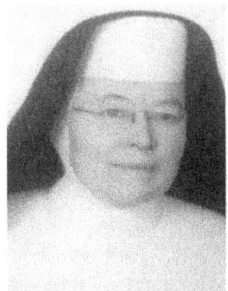

Sister Bernice

Jack tried to describe in his letters, during his first winter away from home, the potent beautiful scent from small white blossoms on orange and grapefruit trees. These trees were everywhere and grown in groves as most of the economy was from ranching and farming. Whenever Jack could catch a ride into the city of Phoenix, he toured the "Valley of the Sun" so called as it is sunny 300 days of the year and surrounded by beautiful mountains. He admired Spanish-style buildings and paved roads completed in the 1920s. Two new organizations in the 1940s were the Phoenix Symphony Orchestra and the Phoenix Art Museum. During WWII, the desert areas in Arizona served as military bases and some personnel chose to remain in Arizona after leaving the service. Many German and Italian prisoners of war chose to stay in Phoenix after 1945 rather than return to their homeland.

The dry heat of Arizona was so helpful to Jack, he became stronger and his lungs improved. His daily walks and mountain climbing seemed to increase his lung volume and he rarely had episodes of wheezing. His physical education instructor at college was a Norwegian man, Coach Lavik; he had Jack run three miles every day. After a year in Arizona Jack improved enough that when he went home for the summer, he passed the military physical for the draft. He traveled to Fort Snelling in St Paul, Minnesota from Moorland and after acceptance into the military; an eye doctor prescribed a pair of eyeglasses. For the first time in his life, Jack could see in the distance clearly and found that on the shooting range he was an excellent shot. He was strong, fit and energetic and developed into a handsome man, especially in a military uniform. He was excited to get on with life, had high self-esteem and was looking forward to whatever came around the corner. Jack traveled to Camp Crowder in the Missouri Ozarks for six weeks of basic training. His dark haired sergeant was a combat veteran, a loud Italian from Chicago who smoked a big cigar. In that photo, Jack knelt down next to him on his right when they took the photo of his platoon after basic training was finished.

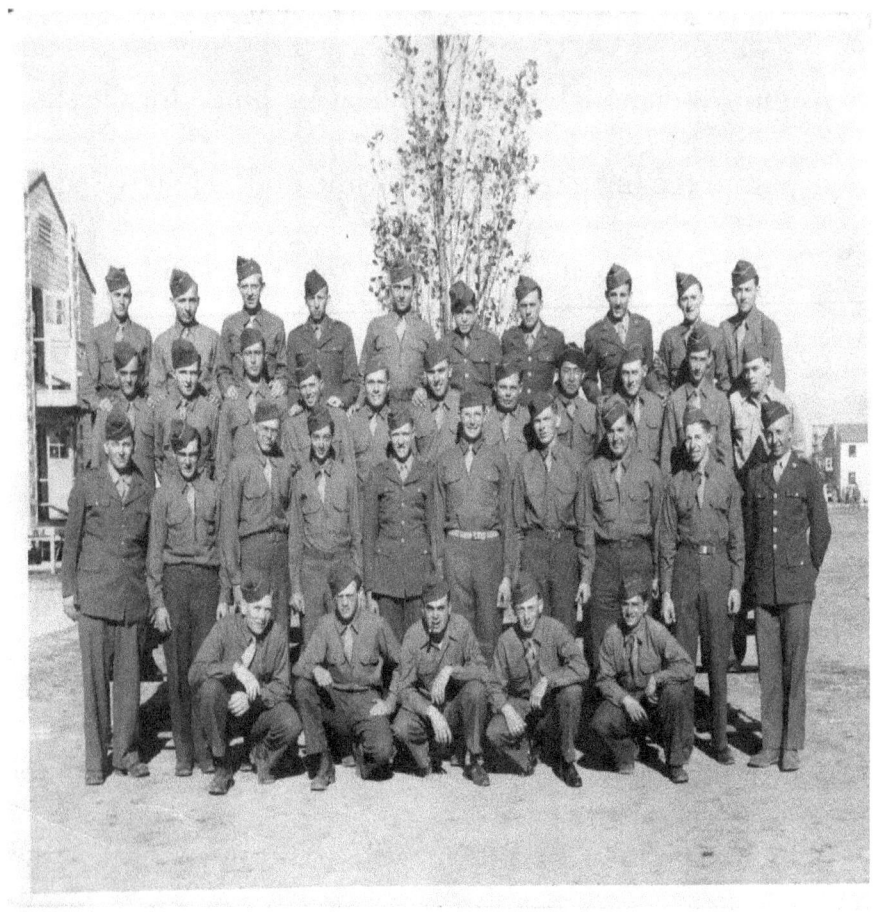

Jack at basic training – first row second from the left

After basic training, Jack went to Fort Sam Houston in San Antonio, Texas where he would spend the next two years. He worked in parasitelogy at Brooke Army Medical Center

(BAMC) and taught others how to use the laboratory. He learned to do blood chemistry, bacteriology and lab work such as the erythrocyte sedimentation rate to detect inflammatory conditions such as rheumatoid arthritis. For the sedimentation rate, he inserted whole blood into a special tube called the Westergren tube. After a certain period of time he would measure how low the erythrocytes or red blood cells settled into the bottom of the tube. The lower they had settled the higher degree of inflammation in the body. People with rheumatoid arthritis had high degrees of inflammation but smokers and obese people had abnormal values also. Jack measured glucose using the folin wu technique and nitrogen in the blood using ammonia solution. He used his microscope daily and loved his job; he spent hours observing bacteria and parasites that he carefully prepared in slides. His favorite lab test was looking for a live spiraling spirochete bacterium called Treponema palladium on a slide he specially stained using a dark field microscope with a special light to illuminate the cause of syphilis. Before penicillin arrived, treatment was with heavy metals such as arsenic or mercury. Syphilis causes behavioral health problems; the most obvious examples of two famous people with the disease are Adolf Hitler and Al Capone. In the future, Jack's favorite laboratory technique would become much simpler- a blood test called the VDRL (Venereal Disease Research Lab) was developed.

Years later Jack returned to Fort Sam Houston and spent time in San Antonio, Texas touring the River Walk area, which did not exist when he had lived there. He stayed at a Fisher House named after a Native American called Powless in Fort Sam Houston to provide emotional support to his daughter Michelle whose husband Tom was undergoing surgery for a cervical injury he received during deployment to Afghanistan for Operation Enduring Freedom after 9/11.

Fisher Houses are a home away from home for the family of the fallen while the soldier recovers. Snacks and water bottles are provided and there were toys and a playground for the children of the injured soldiers. There are computers available for email or Internet access and fresh clothes for injured soldiers just arriving from Germany. Many times worried families would get a phone call about their injured soldier and board a plane to travel to Fort Sam Houston to be with them as soon as possible and not bother to pack a suitcase. Fisher Houses supply housing, clothes, food, phone cards and toiletry items to the worried families whenever necessary. Jack felt immense gratitude when Denzel Washington arrived and, after a tour, wrote out a check for over a million dollars to build an additional Fisher House at Fort Sam Houston. War had been an unpleasant fact for Jack and he knew how important it was to support soldiers and their families.

Jack was amazed at the incredible medical technology and the competent surgical care provided to combat soldiers. He investigated a new burn unit being built right across from where he was staying at the Powless House. After a soldier had surgery or treatment at the hospital, they were able to return to a Fisher House where their families were able to be with them and care for them. However, the hospital was always near. This is a supportive healing environment for these soldiers and their families.

Jack stayed in a room next to his daughter and son in law and joined them at the surgeon's office to discuss Tom's X-rays. The doctor used an electronic health record (EHR) and Jack was amazed at the quality of the X-ray film. When Jack had trained in Fort Sam Houston, he became a medical service corpsman to provide emergency support in the battlefield. He learned how to bandage, splint and administer plasma or morphine. This training provided an overview of the available general practice of medicine known at the time; and on the battlefield, the wounded soldiers referred to these men as "DOC". Jack was never in combat but knew Gene Smith, the husband of his cousin Cecelia Halligan, a distinguished

WWII combat veteran of some terrible battles in the South Pacific. After the war, Gene worked as an orderly in a hospital in Fort Dodge, Iowa in 1946. Medical care at that time allowed him to do just about everything and back then, he did. He was a surgical assistant, worked in the emergency room and provided patient care on the ward. Later, he retired and worked as a barber or a "short robed surgeon". The barber pole of white and red is a symbol of blood and bandages, as barbers long ago would perform minor surgery such as the extraction of teeth and removal of cysts.

Jack was aware his GI bill would pay for college for three years but was concerned about the additional costs not covered for the remaining two years it would take to complete his medical degree. He decided to take the test to become an officer in the U.S. Army, and was proud to receive a very high score. With determination and confidence about his future, he decided to discuss his test results with the Sergeant Major at

Fort Sam Houston at his office. He made his decision to stay in the Army and complete his medical degree within the system. He knew his father was working hard to send his children to college, but Francis had a great many children. Jack entered the office he thought was the Sergeant Major's for officer candidates to discuss his test results. For almost a half an hour, Jack discussed his personal family situation and his desire for a medical degree with an older distinguished man of tall height and thin build. He explained he wanted to become a doctor but the GI bill would not cover the total expenses. Jack finished his discussion and the man smiled, looked directly in his eye and told him to leave the Army as he could tell Jack would not enjoy "peace time politics." He advised him to save his GI bill for the first three years of medical school and borrow for the last senior year.

Jack suddenly realized he was talking to General Wainwright who was the commander of the 4th Army based at

Fort Sam Houston. The General had been a Japanese POW for 3 years after being captured on an island in the Philippines. The then Major General Wainwright had fought a furious defense on the island of Corregidor for over a month and was often on the firing line with his 3500 soldiers. Against all odds, he had held out with his small group on the island and finally surrendered in May of 1942. The month before, against the orders of Wainwright and MacArthur, Major General King had surrendered over 70, 000 American and Filipino soldiers in the WWII Battle of Bataan in the Philippines. These soldiers were forced to march for over a week with hardly any food or water to a prison camp. During this time, almost twenty thousand of these soldiers were beaten and murdered. This war crime of the Japanese became known as the Bataan Death March. Jack had heard his mother's first cousin, a Catholic priest named Father Tom Kane; vividly describe the horrible conditions of the death march as he had been there. Father Kane survived the ordeal and moved to Dallas where he happened to be in the hospital when President Kennedy died. Jack thanked General Wainwright, followed his advice and left the U.S. Army. The General retired and lived in San Antonio, Texas where he died in 1953. He is buried at Arlington National Cemetery.

After Army discharge Jack went back to Arizona for an additional year of premedical and applied to Creighton University in Omaha, Nebraska, where he would finish his last year and start medical school. Francis was happy Jack was attending Creighton as he himself had graduated from high school there. Francis was from a family who was able to afford to send him to a Catholic boarding school, getting a high school degree for a farm boy back then was not common. An eighth grade education was acceptable in those times after a teacher verified student capabilities with a difficult, intense five-hour exam to qualify for graduation.

Although Francis respected Jack's desire to become a doctor he had reservations about a longer, more expensive college degree. Francis made it clear to Jack he would loan him money when necessary and he could pay the money back with interest. However, he would have to work all through college so it would not affect the education of other children in the family. With his prosperity in farming, Francis was able to send three sons to Creighton University in Omaha at the same time. Bernard studied general academics, Bud studied and achieved a degree in accounting and Jack stayed with his pursuit in medicine. They all lived at Mrs.Carrigan's rooming house who was a widow who lived within walking distance from the college. Jack's younger brother Thomas obtained a law degree and move to Casa Grande, Arizona where he has a successful law firm. His sister Mary Catherine became a registered nurse and spent time living with Jack's family in Arizona before she married. Jack's younger brother Stephen later retired in Casa Grande, which is 50 miles south of Phoenix. Stephen has a hobby of building model airplanes for Jack's office and is a talented artist known for his sketches, the one of the family farm being a favorite. Although some of Francis and Catherine's children would move away from the small town of Moorland, they would come back to visit and enjoy a dinner of fresh corn on the cob, pork chops and of course, potatoes.

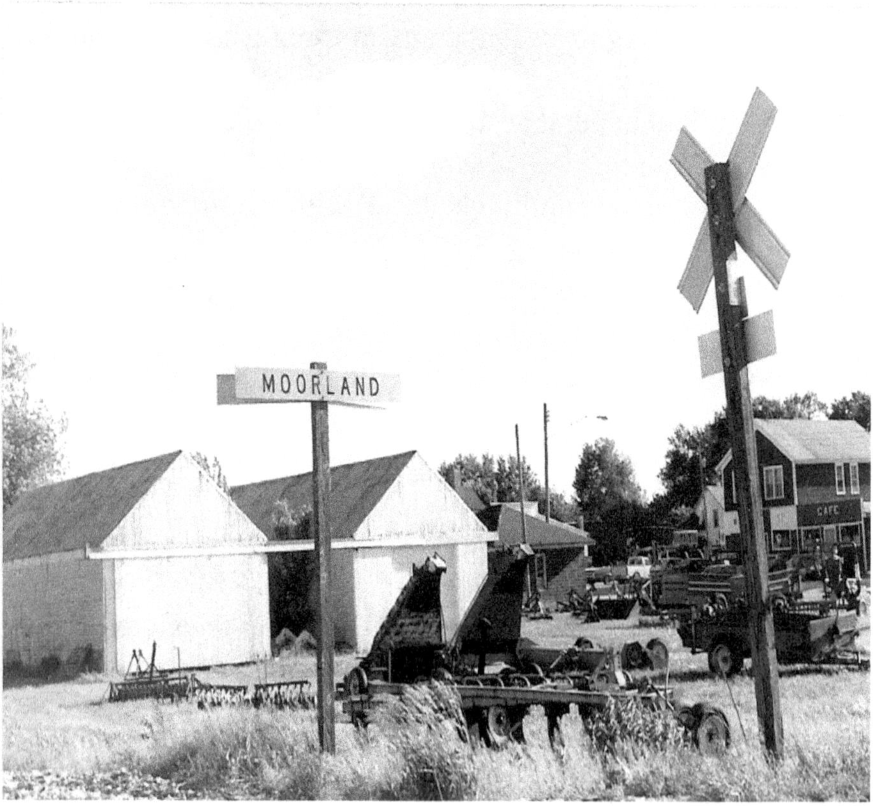

The next year Jack was in his first year of medical school and was able to obtain an apartment living alone for the first time in his life. He had a sense of privacy and the ability to study with no interruptions. He lived in a basement apartment near the college and paid for his monthly rent by stoking the furnace, doing janitorial work and shoveling snow. He had close friendships with some of his classmates who were of better financial status than he was and lived in the fraternity house. These fellow students enjoyed Jack and observed his struggles with finances with obvious amusement. While they attended fraternity parties, Jack would be working hard to provide food or rent for himself. They were amazed when he was unable to afford to buy one important schoolbook required for class, the Grant Atlas of Anatomy. However, he still did well in class. Jack knew he was up against the best and was not afraid to face the fact that he had to work harder to achieve his goal. He may not have had the money or privilege that the fraternity boys did, but he had a fierce determination and graduated with good grades. Jack passed this trait of heightened economy, determination and intelligence on to his children, especially to his second eldest son- Thomas Joseph McCarville who was born in 1954. One day this boy at 17 years of age had twenty dollars in his pocket and was determined to see the City of Los Angeles. He hitchhiked, slept on the beach, ate hot dogs and came home with seven dollars in his pocket. Thomas now is a nuclear scientist and runs a department at the laboratory in Livermore, California testing for anthrax in the environment for homeland security.

Jack went home for the summer of his first year of medical school. His brother Bud was dating a girl named Mary who had a roommate named Marge. Bud organized a double date between Jack and Marge and they dated every summer after that. This same summer Jack worked with his uncle Floyd O'Brien who was married to his mother's sister, Irene Coady. Floyd was a roofer who would buy cedar shingles from the lumberyard and stack them in his truck for the next early morning job. They would climb high up a ladder to the roof on homes, sheds, barns and soon, Jack became a good carpenter. Jack did other work with a first cousin Ray Halligan in the lumberyard making Quonset huts, which were portable wooden rooms the army bought for efficient and quick set up of buildings.

Back at medical school for his second year, Jack enjoyed working as a taxi driver for eight months, but suddenly heard "you are fired!" when he refused to join the teamsters union. He was shocked and surprised when he viewed his overweight boss in his side mirror stomping up to his taxi in a huff, but Jack knew in his heart he was not a "union" man. Still, he was very proud of his smooth driving skills as he could drive with a glass of water on the dashboard of a taxi and never spill a drop. Jack went home to Moorland for the summer after his second year to work for Hormel packinghouse where he wore big plastic gloves to wash bloody tables off after the removal of bones from the hams. He also supervised a large room containing hams sealed in a tin can with gelatin, boiling them in an enormous pressure cooker.

Jack returned to Creighton after the summer to stay in a room at the hospital of St. Catherine's Hospital near the university, and paid for his rent by doing lab work. Before he had left, he asked Marge to marry him. Marge was a beautiful brown-eyed, dark haired bank accountant whose full name was Margaret Yetmar. Her grandfather was from Prague, Czechoslovakia whose name originally having the spelling of Jetmar. The spelling was changed for unknown reasons at the time of his immigration. Her brother Charles is a Catholic priest; their mother is Irish with the name of Margaret Burke. Margaret Burke had a similar childhood to Jack's mother as when she was eight years old, her mother died in childbirth. Father McGuire married Marge and Jack September 8, 1951 at Saint Matthews Church in Clare, Iowa. Marge's sister Arlene was maid of honor and Jack's brother Bud was best man.

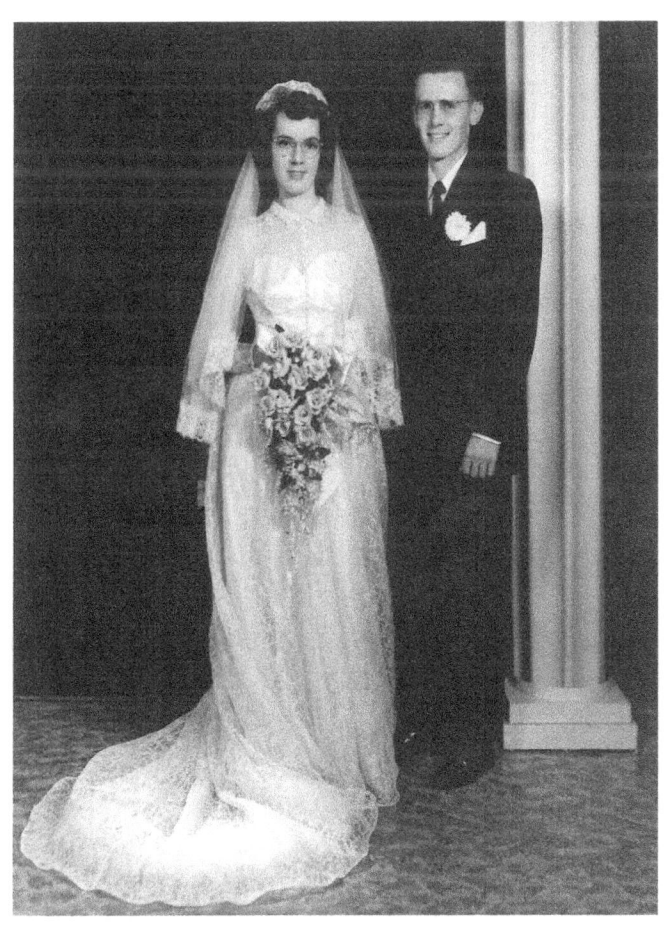

Margaret Yetmar and John Edward McCarville
September 8, 1951

The reception was Marge's home they enjoyed a honeymoon in Minnesota. Marge planned on working at a bank in Omaha during their first year of marriage. The newlyweds moved back to an apartment in Omaha for Jack to complete his final year of school before graduation. Francis wrote up a loan with interest to help the couple live comfortably their first year together. Francis loaned Jack money for living expenses for his last year of school. Their small apartment was an attic with corners that did not allow them to stand up in some areas. A woman with numerous Siamese cats owned the rooming house. One day she asked Jack to spay one of her cats in exchange for rent. The cat had a reaction to the ether and did not survive. Jack paid the rent that month and never attempted to delve into veterinary medicine again. Marge walked and waited at the bus stop every morning to work at a bank job and many times felt the cold and snow unbearable. Most mornings Jack was able to get a lift to school in a car from a fellow student but he often walked home. He always studied hard in the evenings.

As graduation grew near, Jack memorized the Hippocratic Oath, which contains the ethical elements of the practice of medicine to prepare for graduation.

"I do solemnly swear by that which I hold most sacred: That I will be loyal to the profession of medicine, just, and generous to its members; That I will lead my life and practice my art in uprightness and honor; That into whatsoever house I shall enter, it shall be for the good of the sick to the utmost of my power, I holding myself aloof from wrong, from corruption, and from the temptation of others to vice; That I will exercise my art solely for the cure of my patients, and will give no drug, perform no operation for a criminal purpose, even if solicited, for less suggest. That whatsoever I shall see or hear of the lives of men, which are not fitting to be spoken, I will keep inviolably secret. These things I do promise, and in proportion as I am faithful to this, my oath may happiness and good repute be ever mine – the opposite if I shall be for sworn."

Jack graduated from Creighton University School of Medicine in 1952 with a class of 70. Over the years, he had developed a strong friendship with another Irish Catholic in his class named Patrick Phalen, who he would remain close to during his entire career in family medicine. Although Phalen left to specialize at Mayo in Rochester, Minnesota and become a surgeon, he later moved to Phoenix. Patrick used Jack as his assistant surgeon on cases Jack referred to him and if he needed extra help for a surgery. Back then, general practitioners assisted in surgeries but as more physicians specialized, specialists viewed this as inappropriate. Jack and Patrick had similar lives; they were both doctors, Irish Catholic and had large families.

After graduation, Jack and Marge packed their belongings in boxes in preparation to move to Arizona. Marge was excited to move to a warm climate after her winter in Omaha. She was amazed to hear that she would not need a heavy coat during the winter in Phoenix and she would not suffer humidity problems to deal with in the summer.

Money was tight and Jack had to complete one year of internship before he could start his practice as a physician. He applied for his internship in Phoenix at Saint Joseph's Hospital, a Catholic non-profit hospital. One of the doctors Jack knew in Omaha had sold his new yellow Cadillac to a buyer in California and asked Jack and Marge to drive it out there. They packed their boxes in the beautiful car and when they arrived in Los Angeles, they would take a bus to Phoenix. The year of 1952 had deadly outbreaks of tornados and while they were driving in Kansas, the skies turned black and they saw a tornado ahead. They pulled the car over and ran into a restaurant where Jack tried to calm Marge down. Marge was pregnant, terrified of the storm and was vomiting.

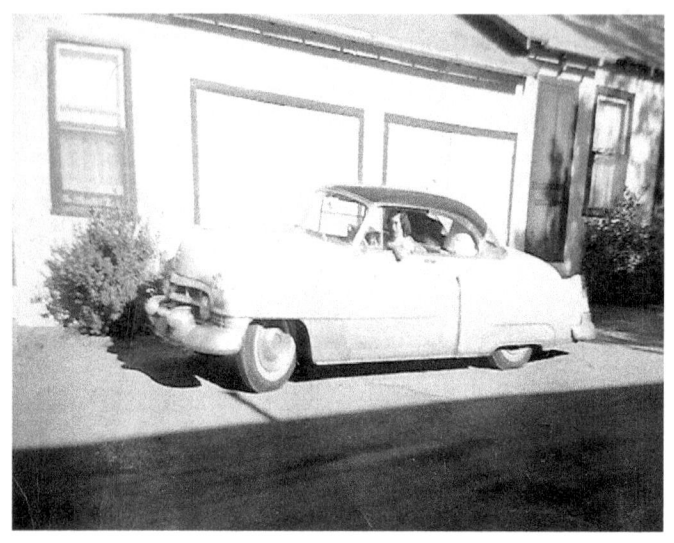

Marge showing off the Cadillac
July 1952

The rest of the trip was smooth and they stopped and mailed their boxes in Las Vegas to the Phoenix post office. When they arrived in California, the buyer of the car drove them to the bus station where they took a bus to Phoenix. Marge sat looking out the windows in awe and Jack smiled when she saw palm trees for the first time. Although they arrived in the summer, the temperature was tolerable. They walked from the Phoenix bus station to a rooming house on 8th avenue and Van Buren- close enough for Jack to walk to work at the hospital. Jack and Marge walked everywhere they needed to go and stayed healthy and fit.

Saint Joseph's Hospital was the first hospital in Phoenix built in 1895 by the Sisters of Mercy. Tuberculosis patients were sent to live in Arizona but after seeing many of these patients die on the streets, the Sisters built a six-room house for them. Years later, they were able to raise money after a Catholic campaign to the community to purchase a dairy farm to build a large hospital on Third Avenue and Thomas. This Catholic, not- for- profit hospital was staffed by the Sisters of Mercy and was where Jack finished his internship. Jack knew that the Sisters were in charge of the hospital although different physicians were assigned to head each floor. The Sisters hired and fired healthcare staff, the floors were spotless and patients received proper care. The Sisters insisted on professional appearance and conduct from everyone including physicians, and supervised every patient's care as if they were a relative. Jack sadly realized later - when the Sisters left the world of healthcare - many other wonderful attributes at the time left with them.

Now, in the United States, one million not-for-profit entities exist and are tax exempt. These include religious, charitable and social welfare as the largest groups and clubs such as war veterans, labor and business leagues. Every interest such as education, arts, culture and religion are involved and in health and human services federal legislation supports social welfare. These not-for-profit organizations have a mission, which is considered a public service rather than moneymaking venture to acquire profit. Not-for-profit entities are able to attract donations by fund raising to acquire buildings and equipment but must use all donations for the public service meant to help maintain its tax-exempt status. Not-for-profit profits are tax-exempt, and file an income tax return to the IRS, Form 990. This is available to the public to view where the for-profit entities are private. Tax-exempt organizations often are exempt from other taxes such as property, sales and state taxes.

The internship Jack completed at Saint Josephs involved rotations through medicine, surgery, pediatrics and obstetrics. The surgeries Jack assisted on were often abdominal surgeries such as appendectomies or hernias with ether drops dripped on a gauze-covered mask for anesthesia. Pediatrics involved mainly respiratory infections with penicillin as an antibiotic and he also helped with the delivery of 10 babies. He was earning 50 dollars a month. Jack ate without charge at the hospital cafeteria and made sure Marge had plenty of fresh food during her pregnancy. They bought fresh eggs from chicken farms and had access to the many orange and grapefruit trees in the area. They enjoyed sampling dates from palm trees that grew over 100 feet high. The farmers had to climb up the trees with special equipment so as not to fall and cover the dates with bags to get the fruit to ripen. Marge became upset when an abundance of horsemeat was for sale as tractors had suddenly replaced horses all over the country. When Patrick Phalen moved to Phoenix, he sold Jack his used car for a few hundred dollars. Jack and Marge enjoyed their first car and the ability to travel around town.

There was a strong fear of polio in the country and vaccines were limited to children. Iron lungs were used to help the patients stricken with polio breathe as they had no strength on their own. The average life span of a man was about 60, Jack and his colleagues considered 60 years old being an "old" man. Jack enjoyed another intern Don Schaler he met while working at Good Samaritan, a large hospital in downtown Phoenix. Don belonged to the U.S. Marine Corps Reserve. He was drafted to Korea as an artillery officer when he was a freshman in medical school. He loves talking about the Howitzer 105 and still does to this day. Don helped develop one of the first prepaid health care plans in Arizona called the Arizona Health Plan. At the time, people did not understand what a prepaid health plan was and Don would try to convince them of the advantages of putting up a deposit and receiving medical care from one organization.

At the end of his internship, Jack was encouraged by one instructor who had been impressed by his expertise in the laboratory to consider specialization in pathology at Mayo Clinic in Rochester. Jack was proud when he obtained the reference for Mayo Clinic from Dr. Stapley who now has a street named after him in Mesa, Arizona. However, Jack made a life changing decision when he became the proud father of his first child, Patrick John McCarville. He knew he needed to start bringing more money into the household. More importantly, Jack knew the cold winters of Minnesota would be hard for Marge to tolerate and he wanted to raise their children in Phoenix. After a great deal of thought, he decided against specialization in pathology and stayed in Phoenix to start a family practice in general medicine. Another instructor Dr. Ovens wrote out a bank reference for Jack to start a general practice and he was able to borrow three thousand dollars from First National Bank. Jack had enough resources to set up an office on 44th Street and Thomas in Phoenix in the Wagon Wheel Shopping Center. He quickly moved his young family to a small rented home nearby.

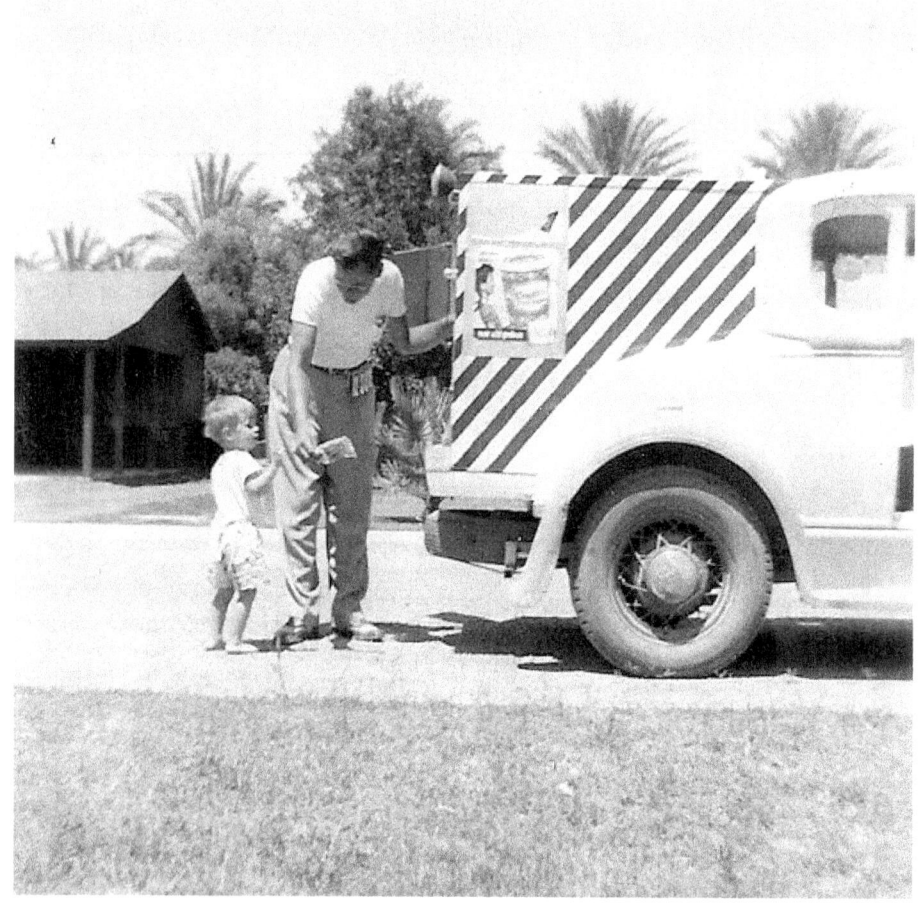

Patrick John McCarville buying ice cream
1953

Jack had a business strategy and placed his office next to a pharmacy owned by a young hard working pharmacist named Glen Crandall. Glen would mop his own floors at night and spent hours making various compounds by hand for prescriptions behind the pharmacy counter. His pharmacy sold cosmetics, cards, and gifts and had a soda fountain with stainless steel equipment, a beautiful grey marble counter and red leather stools. His uniformed staff would make thick malted milk shakes served in tall fluted glasses with whipped cream and a cherry on top. Next to it, they would place the silver metal flask they pulled off from the mixer to refill the glass. The world of retail pharmacy was similar to general practice in medicine as independent businesses were set up by pharmacists who were successful for many years before being taken over by larger corporations.

Jack set up a laboratory in his office with lab equipment he had collected and charged three dollars for an office visit. An elderly woman named Mrs. Anderson volunteered to help him at no charge as she wanted to keep busy and help the young doctor find patients to care for in the area. People slowly started to come from around the neighborhood and local businesses in the area made word of mouth referrals. During Jack's first year of business, there were days he would not see any patients. Sometimes he saw three patients a day. He was concerned about his rent so he paid a hefty sum to have his name "John E. McCarville, M.D." painted on one of the large windows in front of his office. He was surprised when shortly thereafter, the Board of Medical Examiners in Arizona wrote him a letter, ordering him to reduce the size of the lettering as it was too large. During the 1950's ethics in medicine demanded a low-key approach to advertisement. Now physicians are allowed to advertise without restriction and have huge billboards.

    Patients were not asked or expected to pay the three-dollar charge for an office visit on the day of service and most requested a bill to be mailed to their home. Most account receivables were expected to pay within three months and Jack typed the bills himself on a Smith-Corona typewriter. Jack never refused anyone care and neither did the hospitals of Saint Joseph's and Good Samaritan – both of which he was on the staff. The question of how the patient was going to pay the bill was not an issue for medical care at that time. Hospitals would bill an average of 35 dollars a day for a hospital room and extended credit without question. Jack made house calls and carried a bag with him that contained a stethoscope; blood pressure cuff, thermometer, and glass syringes he had previously sterilized in an autoclave at the office. Drugs included vials of penicillin and the narcotic Demerol.

One distressful house call came from a frantic mother who found her baby dead in the crib. With the baby, Jack found a plastic bag the mother had used from the dry cleaners to keep the mattress from becoming wet. Jack realized the child must have had the bag over the mouth and nostril area and died from suffocation. Jack became alarmed as just recently, in the emergency room, he observed another death attributed to this same type of incident. Another baby in a crib had died from the exact same cause. He alerted the police, discussed the danger of using these bags in a crib and the warning was printed in the city newspaper. Suddenly a group of lawyers from Philadelphia from a dry cleaning business challenged his theory. The Center for Disease Control (CDC) investigated the claim and found 72 cases of suffocation resulting from dry cleaner bags. Jack received the Distinguished Community Service Award in January of 1960 from the Maricopa Medical Society for alerting the nation on the dangers of suffocation from plastic bags. A printed warning was placed on all dry cleaner and plastic bags and still exists today.

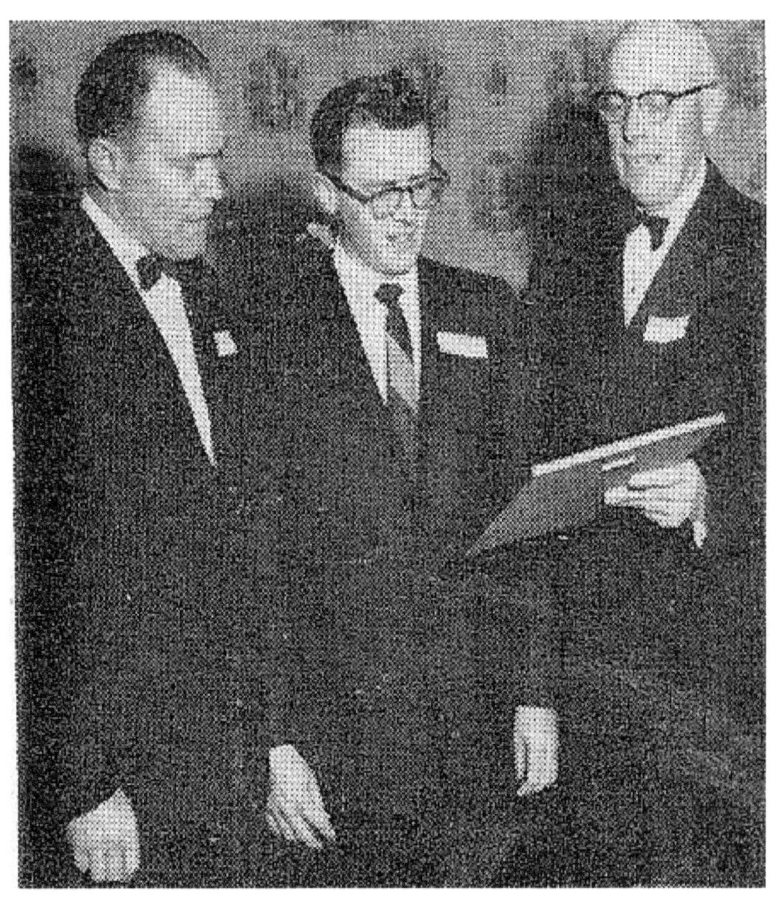

Jack (middle) receiving his award in 1960 for alerting the nation of the dangers of suffocation from plastic bags.

Jack was in the U.S. Army Reserves, as the military required physicians to do so in case they must call upon him for duty. This was known as the "Doctors' Draft." This regulation was in place from the 1950s and did not end until the early 1970s to the dismay of most physicians who could be drafted if needed for war. Personally, Jack never was concerned about the regulation as he enjoyed his time with the military and viewed life as a never-ending adventure. While in the Army Reserves, he examined new recruits on his mandatory reserve days, which included checking their urine for protein and sugar, and acuity of their vision. One young recruit could not read the letters on the vision chart. Jack realized it was because he could not read and so, he did not pass him as all recruits had to read and write. Jack met and examined many soldiers on his reserve days and was able to ride in various aircraft - his favorite being helicopters. His eldest son Patrick John McCarville became a helicopter pilot after being drafted and made his career in aviation, retiring as a colonel. While all the pilots Jack examined enjoyed him as their doctor, he in turn enjoyed caring for physically fit young men after spending a day in his office caring for the sick.

During his first year of practice, Jack built up a positive amount of account receivables with office visits and house calls but payments were very slow coming in. He decided to improve cash flow by working nights at the city jail. He earned five dollars a night examining prisoners with health complaints and if they needed hospitalization, he admitted them to the Maricopa County Hospital on 24th Street and Roosevelt in Phoenix, which had jail beds. He soon became familiar with one frequent prisoner, Ira Hayes, a famous Native American war veteran born on the Gila River Indian Reservation. Ira was the first soldier Jack took care of in his career who suffered from the effects of war, now called post-traumatic stress disorder or PTSD. Ira was in jail most Saturday nights after drinking at a bar on Washington Street in Phoenix that was the closest in proximity to his reservation. Jack later realized the Irish are similar to Native Americans; it is much wiser for the Irish and the Indian not to drink. Ira Hamilton Hayes was a handsome, intelligent man with a unique sense of humor and Jack was sad to learn of his death at the early age of 32 years in January of 1955 on his reservation. Ira enlisted in the Marines in 1942 and in 1945 became part of a photographic flag rising at Iwo Jima that would symbolize the valor and patriotism of World War II. During World War I, many Native American Indians entered the military service though they were not required to do so if they were living on a reservation. In World War II, Native Americans were drafted and joined units made up mainly of Caucasians. After the war, many of them returned to their reservations Phoenix has one of the largest concentrations of Native Americans in the United States. Like Ira Hayes, Jack found Native Americans have a unique sense of humor. Jack once asked a Navajo patient to teach him to say, "Hello, how are you?" in Navajo but found out later by another Navajo patient he had been taught to say, "Your ass is on fire!"

Jack had Spanish patients and wanted to learn their language as well as Arizona is close to the Mexico border and midway between Los Angeles, California and El Paso, Texas. He signed up for a Spanish class on the central west side of town in a community college called Phoenix College. One afternoon on his way to class, he met a man who would change his life forever. Darrel Sawyer was offering flying lessons at five dollars an hour. These lessons were available from a company called Phoenix Flight School which had six instructors. Jack struggled with the cost of these classes but felt the risk was a good opportunity for the future. He knew some physicians who flew to work in towns that were in need of physicians. Jack attended classes at Sky Harbor Airport. Then one day a week for three months Jack went to ground school. After ground school he flew with an instructor for dual instruction for 10 hours in a plane called an Aero Champ. This plane has two central wheels and a small tail wheel. He had to fly solo in the plane with an accurate take off and short flight around the airport ending in a proper landing. Jack enjoyed every minute of his classes and his flights out of Sky Harbor.

Minutes before his solo flight, he could hardly contain his excitement. After checking the plane to make sure it was in proper working order, he started the engine with help from his instructor who turned the propeller blade on the front engine. It started after two attempts and he turned the small plane and directed it to the runway. Looking straight ahead, he lined himself up and pulled the steering handle slowly toward him. He reached full power with the noise and vibration humming in his ears and began barreling down the runway. With a grip of steel, he steered with intense concentration down the middle of the runway, slowly and gently lifting off the ground in a smooth exhilarating rush upward. He realized he was utterly alone in the aircraft when he had reached his designated altitude. He could not believe what he had just accomplished! Fighting back the tears in his eyes, he congratulated himself for a second and then concentrated fully on his flight of independence and freedom from the instructor. He suddenly hit air pockets that jolted him upward in his seat but he knew from his previous experiences those were normal and nothing to fear. He relaxed after the plane settled and for a quiet moment, he looked outward then down, and enjoyed the sights he was able to see below on this beautiful day. Phoenix has many mountains, one is Camelback named because it resembled the shape of a camel, and another he could see at the same time was Squaw Peak, the name newly changed to Piestewa Peak. In addition, he could see the famous Superstitions, mountains with stories of lost gold treasure and South Mountain. Phoenix in the air appears to be sectioned off in squares, making it easy to navigate.

Jack had to land next and centered the plane toward the middle of the runway. He was able to guide the plane toward the ground without a jolt, making a perfect landing. Happy to be back on land safely, he turned the plane into the designated parking place near the hanger and stopped the engine. He sat back in an exhausted heap and thought it was over, that was it. His flight had been a birth of power, exhilaration and strength with bumps, sudden jolts up and down, then a gradual descent toward a sudden stop, which ended it all. Jack realized the cycle of life is very similar to that of a plane flight.

After a few years of flying, Jack bought a Tri- Pacer, which has a nose wheel; the three wheels of the plane together resemble a tricycle. Jack often flew to Payson to work at a clinic that did not have a physician and flew over the skies of Phoenix every weekend with his family and friends. His growing family became used to jumping in the car and driving to Sky Harbor where they parked the car near the lone control tower after crossing railroad tracks. They waited patiently for their father and played with the kittens near the hanger as he carefully prepared the plane. One kitten of particular interest had lost the tips of his ears from being too close to a propeller during start up. All the children took turns sitting up front and the lucky one was always overjoyed to be the one to pretend to "fly" the plane with their father. Jack would never tire of explaining the instrument panel and showing his children how he aligned the wings of the plane horizontally in one of the gauges.

Jack flew two trips to Iowa with Marge and their four young children, Patrick, Michelle, Thomas and Zita. Jack encouraged Marge to take flying lessons and she flew her solo but never had the passion for flying that Jack did. On one trip out of town, she was seen hanging up wet diapers to dry on the wings of their plane. One special trip Jack took was to La Paz, Mexico with his father-in-law John Yetmar who caught a large tuna, which really made his day, as he was an avid fisherman. Whenever Jack and Marge's parents came out to Arizona together to visit in 1953 and were amazed at the beauty of the desert.

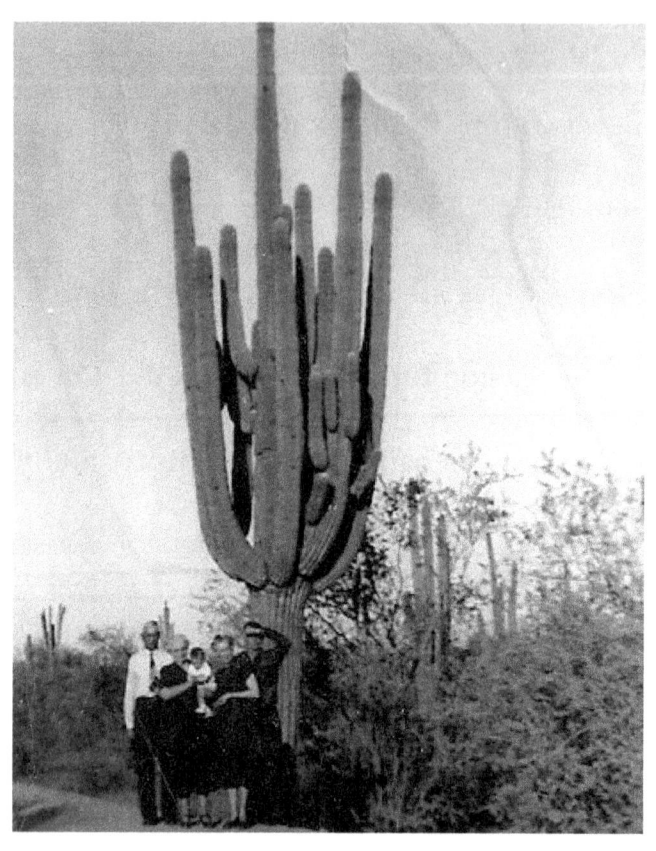

John Yetmar, Margaret Yemar, Patrick John McCarville, Catherine McCarville and Francis McCarville enjoying the Arizona desert, 1953.

One year Jack rented a biplane called a Steerman, which were used as primary trainers in World War II before they were phased out. Soon they became popular as crop dusters and stunt planes. Jack used the plane to teach himself to do rolls and stalls. Marge never understood why Jack had no fear that he would leave his children without a father while he was teaching himself to fly in this manner.

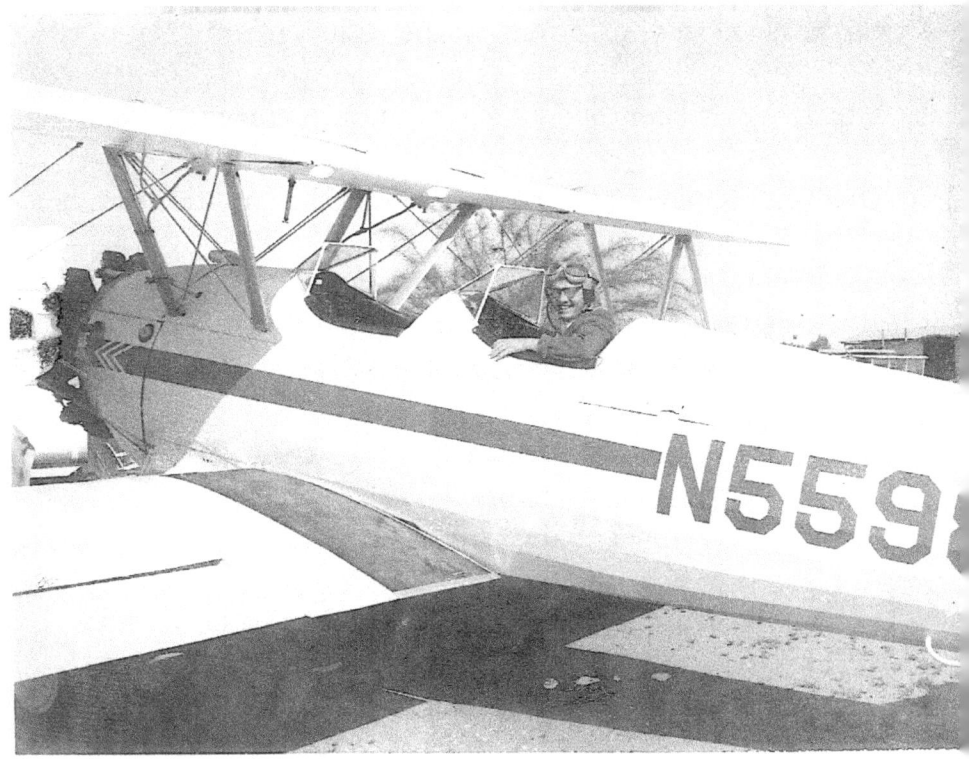

Jack in a Steerman

Jack performed many flight physicals at the Arizona Army National Guard as a FAA Medical Examiner, which any general practitioner could do, but was restricted to certification of medical licenses for third class pilots. In July of 1960 after formal instruction in Oklahoma, he became a Second Class Aviation Medical Examiner due to the large amount of flight physicals he was performing at the Arizona Army National Guard. Years later the Federal Aviation Agency in Oklahoma changed his career as a physician when they notified him he qualified to attend instruction in Alabama to become a First Class FAA Medical Examiner. This was a turning point in his career as now he could devote all of his attention to aviation medicine. He now could certify medical licenses of first class pilots who flew for the airlines. Jack always had a spiritual view of flying. Once he asked his daughter Michelle, "How can anyone say there is not a God?" as they were flying together above the clouds and looking down at it all.

Chapter Five

Modern medicine in America today often requires patients to see a different specialist for each medical condition. If a patient has a stomach disorder but is also having bladder problems, a variety of different specialists will treat the patient. Proper communication between these different physicians may be slow at times and specialists stay in their unique but narrow field. When Jack treated his patients during his early years of general practice, he had the capability, knowledge and skill to treat a variety of conditions in his office where now these patients would be referred to specialists.

Jack's patients did not hesitate to call on him at any time. He made house calls every night and many times Marge and his children came with him – while waiting out in the car in front of the house. Jack was an expert at the stethoscope. He would listen to the five lobes of the lungs and was able to diagnose whether it was congestion or worse, pneumonia. He admitted children with pneumonia to the hospital where they would sleep in a crib under a tent draped with oxygen filtered in. Jack gave penicillin injections in glass syringes sterilized in the autoclave. He gave gold injections for arthritis and the vial contained real gold settled at the bottom.

Jack delivered over 500 babies and one day he even delivered three different babies in one day. He bought an X-ray machine, charged 10 dollars for one X-ray and developed his own films in a small dark room he painted black. This room held three large rinsing trays and he became an expert when to stop rinsing in order to obtain the best quality film. He was able to diagnose many different problems with the X-ray machine such as broken bones and foreign objects. Once a patient stepped on a needle and Jack was able to judge exactly where it was to remove it. He could diagnose pneumonia, emphysema and congestive heart failure which showed fluid in the lung. On rare occasion, a patient would complain of chest pain and the X-ray would show a tumor in the lung area. Jack referred these cases out to a surgeon. He became an expert at the different types of bone fractures, such as a spiral fracture and would sit down with his patients and explain the diagnostics of the X-ray to them. He set bone fractures in a large room in his office using white plaster of Paris casts over Kerlix gauze wraps. After the bone healed, he would remove the cast with a special saw. After a period of time, Jack noticed his own toes were turning brown at the tips from the radiation of the X-ray machine and he purchased a lead apron for protection.

Jack performed sigmoid scopes in the office as well as pap smears and did various minor surgeries such as removal of hemorrhoids, ganglions or sebaceous cysts. He spun down urines for diagnosis of urinary tract infections under the microscope that revealed various bacteria. He prepared slides to diagnose pelvic infections such as yeast or vaginal parasites called trichomonis; these were seen moving quickly about in the saline prep he used on the glass slide. Jack provided almost all aspects of medical care for an individual family. His patients were able to discuss behavioral health issues or marriage counseling. He mentioned to Marge one night he found it "easier to fix a bone than a brain."

If it were necessary for his patient to go to a hospital they could discuss what hospital they wanted to use and what specialists Jack recommended for surgery. Patients were in control of their health care decisions and what provider or organization to use. General practitioners billed patients directly for their medical services and the American Medical Association was opposed to any form of non-physician control over medical professionals. When Jack's patients did need surgery such as an appendectomy, he was able to be the assistant surgeon at the hospital. He would follow their care with visits to the hospital and his familiar face and reassurance during their surgery and postoperative care made a positive impact on their progress.

Some families had insurance coverage for hospital stays as a benefit from their employers. During World War II, the government controlled wages that employers paid their employees. Employers had to compete against each other for employees but wages were fixed. In the 1940s, health insurance evolved as a new idea to attract workers and became a benefit that was soon expected and demanded. This benefit developed into the employer based system we now know today. The Internal Revenue Service issued a ruling in 1943, codified in section 106 of the Code allowing employers to offer employment based health insurance coverage to employees on a tax-free basis. Employees may purchase health benefits through employers with pre-tax dollars. Employers may deduct employer contributions to purchase group health benefits as ordinary and necessary business expenses under section 162 of the Code. Unfortunately, this system will not work with unemployment or catastrophic illness. In addition, employers are in business to make money. Cutting costs by lowering quality of medical insurance policies for their employees can increase the profits in a business.

Sometimes the patients Jack treated did not have jobs and or were uninsured, such as the elderly or poor. When they needed care or hospitalization, he did not charge them for his services. His profession obligated him to serve those too poor to pay. In 1960, there were 16 million people over the age of 65 and social security checks were an average of 72 dollars a month. The government stepped in to help these two populations of elderly and poor in 1965 when Lyndon B. Johnson passed legislation to sign the Medicare bill into law. The law of Medicare pays for the aged over 65 and Medicaid helps the poor. Jack approved of this law but in addition, felt the purpose of the government in medicine should also cover catastrophic loss. Much later in his medical career, he would realize that medical insurance became necessary to cover the enormous cost of the advances of modern technology in healthcare.

Jack documented his patient's visits by hand and kept them organized alphabetically in manila folders. He graduated to using a recording device called a stenograph that he talked into and he paid for a service where staff would collect the colorful tapes, listen to them and type them. He once had a secretary who took short hand and typed his notes from that. He filed his records in large three drawer filing cabinets and used a typewriter to type letters for correspondence. He hired a CPA to manage his taxes and bought a large salt-water aquarium and magazine subscriptions for his waiting room. Jack enjoyed family life and church activities at Saint Thomas the Apostle and stayed active in the Civitan Club, selling fruitcake at Christmas to promote citizenship. Every year before Christmas he packed a large box of food and together with his wife and kids in the station wagon delivered the box to a needy family he knew needed help. Jack and Marge loved President Kennedy and were thrilled when he had visited Phoenix as a Senator in 1960. They especially enjoyed following the news when he visited his ancestors home in Ireland in 1962.

Marge was always active in the church, especially with activities for the poor. Marge kept in close contact with her family in Iowa and convinced her sister Arlene to move out to the nearby town of Scottsdale, Arizona. Arlene had severe asthma and Marge knew the hot dry climate would be much better for her health. Arlene was married to John Heun and they would have eleven children. Birth control was not an option for devout Catholic women and the stress of the constant pregnancies was very difficult for the two sisters. Although Marge may have been pregnant most of the time, she still enjoyed going out on the town at night with Jack to the music and dance clubs in Phoenix. They collected their favorite music on vinyl records to include Frank Sinatra and Roger Miller. Jack often sang "King of the Road" or "Mack the Knife" but his favorite music was Marty Robbins.

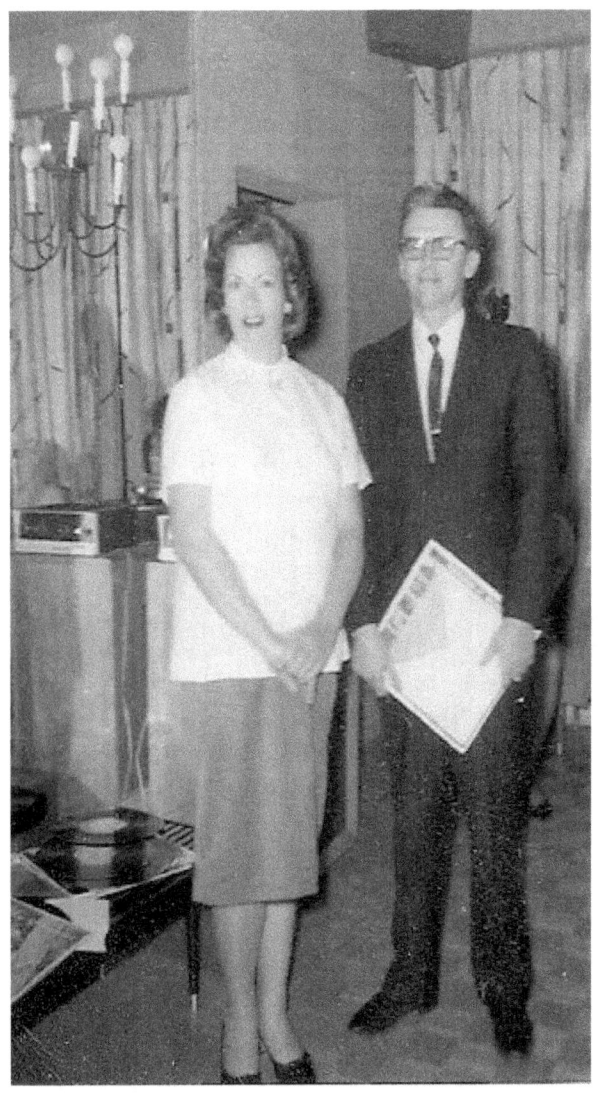

Jack and Marge adding to their vinyl record collection in 1964

Everyone in the family remembers the special day when Jack brought home a new and novel item - a television console. His children would sit on the floor enjoying the Wallace and Ladmo Show and once, a British band called the Beatles on The Ed Sullivan Show. They had an Australian Shepherd dog they named Pokey and they all danced frantically to a vinyl record called The Monster Mash. Jack always wore a white shirt, black pants and tie to the office. After a difficult day, he drank Alka Seltzer while enjoying his new TV and had his own special private time watching Johnny Carson late into the evening. If one of Jack's many children woke up during this time they knew they could join their father in his TV chair and go back to sleep in his arms.

Jack and Marge enjoyed their dance lessons together and did well in the Arthur Murray Dance Studio competitions, a few they attended were out of state. Marge often wore elaborate dresses during a competition and Jack dressed to match his dance instructor who chose their costume to match the music. Jack bought Marge a fur coat and after lessons, they would often eat at a restaurant near the studio, the Green Gables on 24th Street and Thomas. This was built to appear as a castle with a man dressed as a knight on a large white horse who greets their car at the gate. Two restaurant's on Central Avenue in Phoenix Jack and Marge often went to were a steakhouse called Durant's where they entered through the kitchen and Macayo's a Mexican food restaurant. In the 1960's high school kids on Fridays after a football game who had a high performance vehicle or "muscle car" would drive slowing down Central Avenue showing off their car to other teenagers who gathered there to hang out. Jack and Marge enjoyed going to the Phoenix Symphony especially during the Christmas season. Sometimes they would go to the horse races at Turf Paradise or the dog races at Phoenix Greyhound Park but Marge remembers they never won anything.

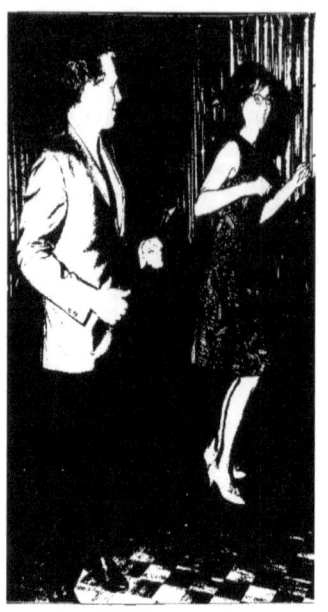
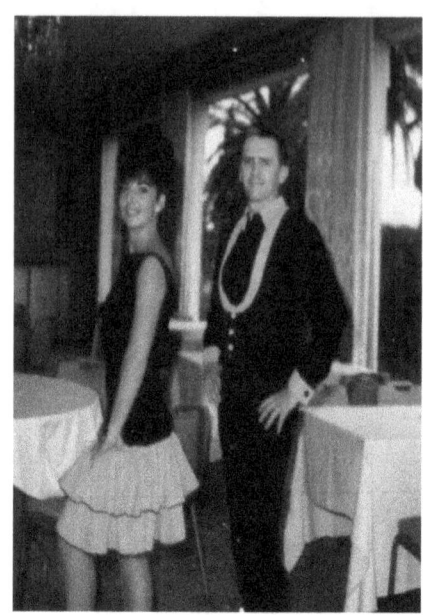

Jack in various dance competitions in the Arthur Murray Dance Studio with his dance instructors

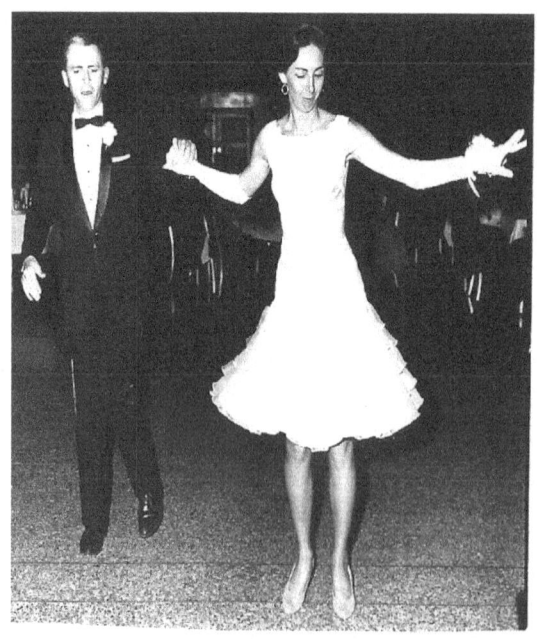

The family loved to jump in their station wagon and ride to Bob's Big Boy for the novel idea of a drive-in restaurant where a server would take their hamburger orders from the car. Many times on Saturdays in the summer, they would go to the Round-Up Drive In to watch a movie. Each car was charged one dollar and the children would run to the family playground right in front of the movie screen. Seats were available near the playground and a snack bar was near the restrooms. The children would buy Big Hunks, Cracker Jack, Sweet Tarts, and Candy Cigarettes. People smoked everywhere and children drove around in cars that had no seat belts. Whenever families packed up to leave the drive- in after the movie, someone was always heard shouting after they broke their car window out from the force of the metal speaker they forgot to remove from the car before driving away.

Marge was thrilled when Jack built up enough funds to build a custom home. Marge and Jack designed a home that had air conditioning, three bathrooms, three bedrooms, and large kitchen with laundry room, family room with wood burning fireplace, living room and dining room. They had a huge back yard for the children with many orange, grapefruit and palm trees. Jack bought a boat to enjoy trips to the many lakes around Phoenix such as Roosevelt, Pleasant and Saguaro Lake. Most of the children learned how to water ski and fish, and sons Patrick and Mark later became tournament fishermen. Sundays after Mass, Jack would often take the family to the Ramada Inn on Van Buren and rent out a room for the day so he could teach them how to swim in the hotel pool. The large family of five boys and three girls enjoyed a restaurant near there, Bill Johnson's Big Apple, which had sawdust on the floor. The servers were dressed as cowgirls with a gun in their gun belts. Marge drove a green Suburban to transport the children to Saint Thomas the Apostle

Elementary School and Jack coached little league baseball.

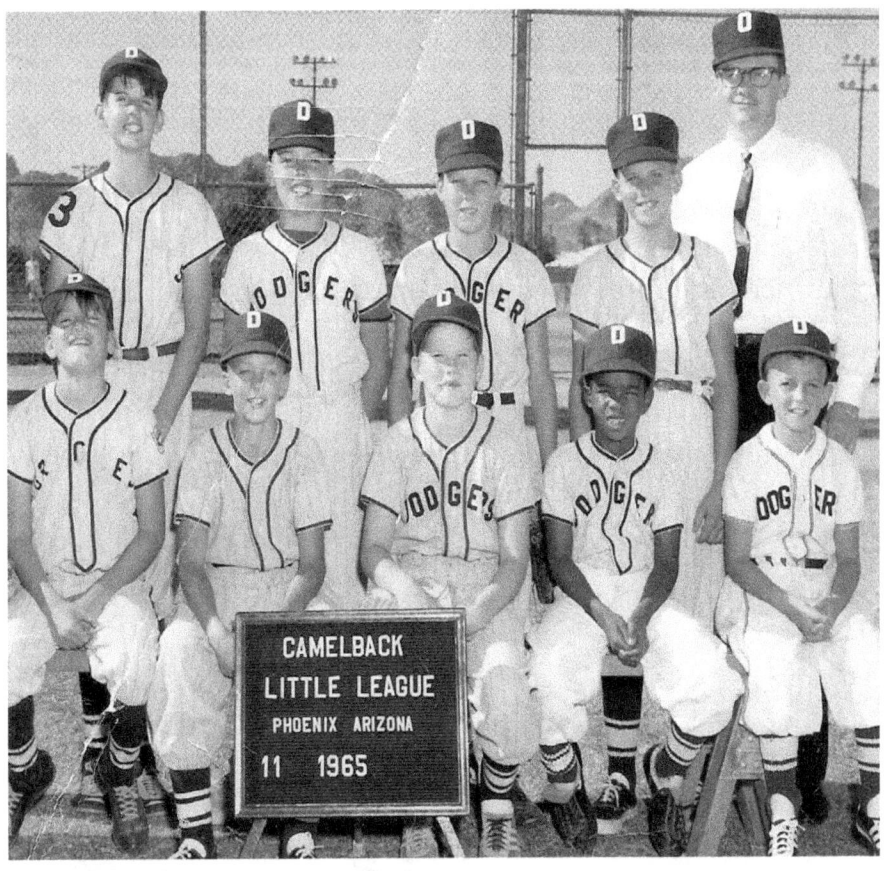

Patrick John McCarville top left, Thomas Joseph McCarville bottom left, Jack top right, 1965

Jack and Marge would be proud of the education and careers their eight children would have. Patrick John and Francis Xavier would spend time in the Army with their careers to be in aviation. Thomas Joseph and William Charles would become engineers with specializations in defense and aerospace. Mary Michele, Zita Marie and Ann would have careers in pharmacy and nursing. Mark Edward, who has the genetic Black Irish trait of premature grey hair, was a detective for the Tempe police department. He retired from the police department and after intensive training, he now practices as a specialist in pediatric cardiac ultrasound.

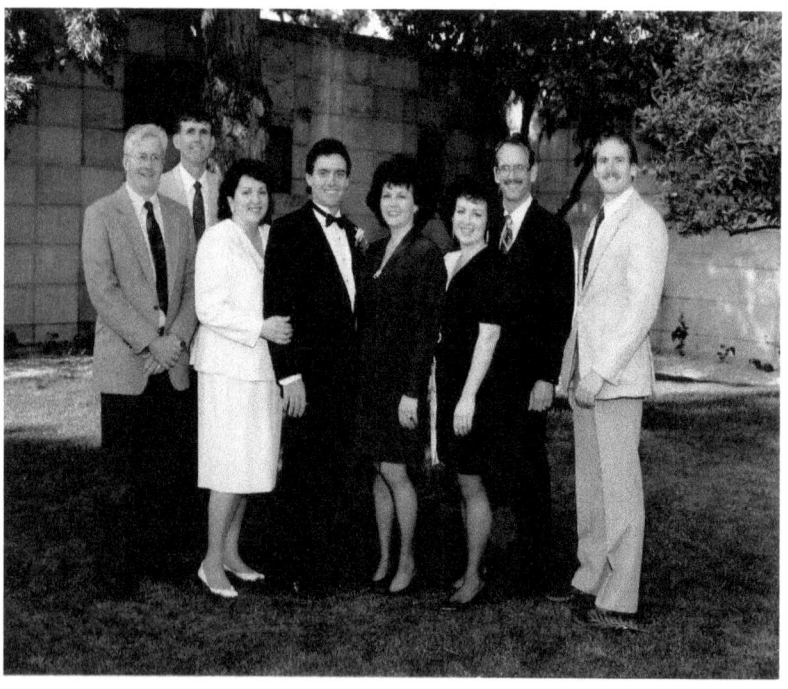

Mark Edward McCarville, Patrick John McCarville, Zita Marie McCarville, William Charles McCarville, Mary Michele McCarville, Anne McCarville, Francis Xavier McCarville, Thomas Joseph McCarville

Jack felt standards were necessary for all physicians to make care available at reasonable fees; he had been that taught that greed must not enter into the profession of medicine. Before Medicare, patients did not seek out healthcare until necessary but with Medicare, doctor visits began to increase. Suddenly elective surgeries were being asked for and a boom in these procedures, especially for specialists became dramatic. For instance, when ophthalmologists accepted assignment that is, took whatever Medicare paid as full payment for cataract surgery, their offices were suddenly filled to capacity with elderly patients demanding the elective surgery. This outrageous consumer demand of Medicare was completely unexpected by the government. Jack and other medical professionals soon realized that the billing of Medicare and Medicaid was out of control. Five years after the Medicare law passed, the government had paid over 60 million claims totaling more than 18 billion dollars.

Besides patients wanting to use insurance to obtain services, there was no limit on physician charges or the amount of profit for services. The enormous prices soon came under scrutiny, and regulations began to emerge to control unnecessary tests and define appropriate procedures for a certain diagnosis. After Medicare began in 1965, spending rose rapidly within the "fee-for-service" delivery system, as physicians were free to increase both their charges and the volume of service they provided. The lure of huge profits by providers and hospitals alike increased the number of patients receiving services with no limit on the services they received. To compound the problem of increased services and number of patients, the 1970's healthcare costs in Medicare had unexpected high expenditures because of advances in technology and medications. This, combined with rapid inflation and exploitation of the fee-for-service system, threatened the very solvency of Medicare.

The first strategy to control Medicare expenditures was legislation by frantic policymakers to restrain fees. In 1972, a mandate on the yearly increase in physicians' fees was limited to the Medicare Economic Index or MEI. This attempt at control was to limit the growth of fees alone. Providers were not willing to give up their high profits and responded by increasing their volume of services. Costs continued to rise throughout the 1980s. The government attempted a second strategy in 1984 called the Deficit Reduction Act or DEFRA. This act "froze" physician fees and established a Participating Physicians Program. This program paid a participating physician who signed up with the program, 80 percent of the determined fee schedule of Medicare for a service as total payment for the service. They were not allowed to bill the patient the remaining 20 percent called balance billing. A nonparticipating physician would be paid 76 percent of the fee schedule but would be allowed to participate in balance billing and bill the patient the remainder of the original charge. This caused a high remainder amount for the patient to pay to nonparticipating physicians. The previous problem of physicians increasing patient volume continued to increase the total costs in Medicare. Limits of the rise in fees alone without concern for the volume of services proved ineffective in controlling expenditures.

Another change after the implementation of Medicare was increased specialization of physicians. Jack started to hear complaints from patients when they could not request him to provide services in the hospital. Specialization of physicians discontinued the use of general practitioners to follow their referral patients in hospital care. Now that Medicare or other insurance was available to pay medical bills, family members worried about a loved one who would insist they see "a specialist". A diagnosis from Jack would result in a referral to a specialist who would take over that particular region of care. Jack would refer out his surgical cases such as appendicitis and no longer assist in the surgery or perform postoperative care.

Specialists would seek Jack out to increase their referral base and send gifts at Christmas. Sometimes Jack did not have to pay for medical care from specialists his children needed. For example, a visit to the ophthalmologist for glasses for the children was "no charge" as Jack would refer cataract patients to them. Patrick Phalen, pictured below on the left in 1960, used Jack to assist in his surgeries until specialists took over.

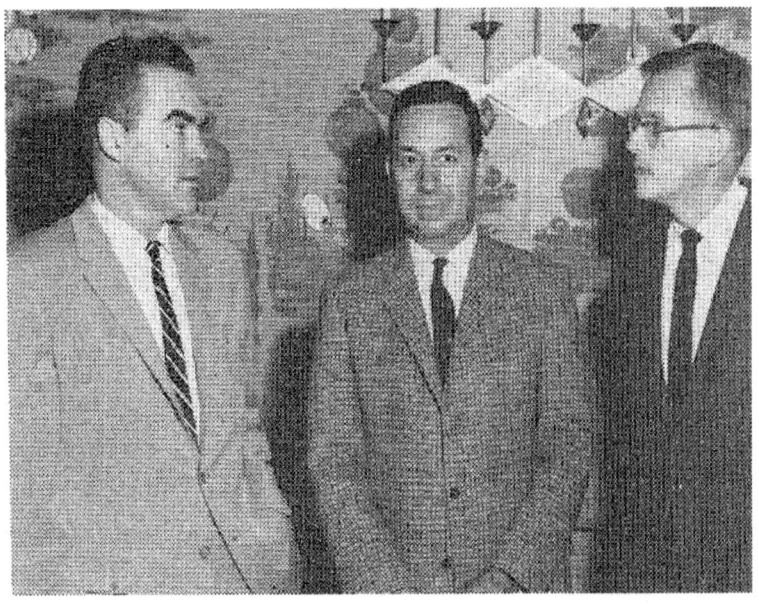

During this time, a difference in pay between the general practitioner and the specialist became dramatic. Medical students began to realize early on, if they went into family practice, their salary would be much lower and office hours longer than if they were to specialize. A specialist could make more than double the amount of a family provider and medical students have a large debt, so money was a serious issue. Malpractice insurance evolved as different specialties in medicine grew. When insurance for obstetrics rose to $30,000 per year, Jack stopped delivering babies.

Patients became capable of increasing the cost of healthcare when they found a lawsuit against a physician would prompt the insurance company to settle for a quick $100,000 out of court to avoid litigation. This was without any decision of who was wrong in the first place. Malpractice rates skyrocketed and physicians responded to the increase in malpractice suits by increasing prices and decreasing the amount of time they spent with each patient. Quick visits at a higher price with an increase in volume increased profit margins. Physicians began to practice in a defensive, cautious manner spending time and efforts on meticulous documentation. Tests were ordered to improve documentation in the event of a malpractice lawsuit in the future. This additional cost of documentation drove up the price of healthcare.

Jack realized the Hippocratic Oath to which he had so proudly sworn on the day of his graduation took a back seat to profits. The business of caring became a business for profit. Gradually, new medical graduates were administered a new modified version of the Oath to keep up with the changes in medical practice. A new idea to control hospital costs began in New Jersey in 1980, converting the existing hospital reimbursement system with a Diagnosis Related Group or "DRG-based" payer system. Yale researchers developed the DRG system, which simply is a pricing for the top one hundred common inpatient hospital procedures, such as appendectomy or hysterectomy. The concept of DRG payments is that they are fixed and paid based on the patient diagnosis. DRG payments have no regard for the actual costs of the hospital. For instance, a hospital would be paid a set fee of $2,000 for removal of a gallbladder no matter what waste the nurse or doctor caused for the procedure or how many days the patient stayed in the hospital. For the first time, incentives developed for hospitals to become cost-effective. If the hospitals did not manage cost, there was no method to be reimbursed for their losses. Patients suddenly began to leave the hospitals very early after surgical procedures; they were escorted to the family car with family members in shock who complained their loved ones were leaving the hospital too soon. Many times the family members concern was correct as elderly spouses unable to care for their partners, would have to be readmitted to the hospital- but now under a new DRG. This new DRG would pay for the new hospital stay but still did not make up for the trauma of the previous discharge that was too early for the patient's family to handle. However, the DRG system worked. The DRG system was able to start controlling hospital spending but physicians were not affected by this new hospital system.

Gradually, the success of the DRG payment system in the hospital began to enter other healthcare businesses. Under President Reagan, hospitals began to shift payments to diagnosis (DRG) rather than by treatment. Medicare shifted to this system and private healthcare corporations began to follow the system. Insurance companies kept complaining that the physicians were exploiting the fee for service system of payment. Under President Nixon, federal legislation began to provide assistance to prepaid healthcare plans, which were renamed Health Maintenance Organization (HMO).

Medicare tried a third strategy in January of 1992 to restrain growth of Medicare spending for physician services with the implementation of a physician fee schedule called Medicare Fee Schedule. Providers simply increased their patient load and patients started to feel they were just a number when in a doctor office. The effort to control the problem of volume by physicians was called the Sustainable Growth Rated or SGR in 1998. Patients were shocked when the effect of those reductions caused physicians to drop Medicare patients; patients found no Medicare providers available and lost access to health care services. This led to the development of the Medicare Modernization Act stepping in to allow increases in payments.

Jack continued general practice while observing the astonishing change in the payment systems in healthcare. The payment system was changing from Medicaid, Medicare, Blue Cross, Commercial (that paid 100% of gross charges) and self-pay to HMO, PPO and capitated arrangements. Jack was amazed to see insurance companies having the power to choose a consumer's physician and, if the patient was in need of a specialist, an authorization was required from the insurance company that would choose the specialist. With PPO or Preferred Provider Organizations, the insurance company developed a range of network providers that was less restrictive than the HMO. Authorizations by the insurance company were not required as long as the provider was within the network of insurance company approved providers. With capitated insurance plans, a monthly fee similar to car insurance premiums is required and healthcare is available on an as needed basis.

Jack continued his work as a physician with the Arizona Army National Guard at the Papago Park Military Reservation near the Phoenix Zoo on 56th Street and McDowell in Phoenix. His duties included medical exams on reservists and pilots. He extended his expertise in aviation medicine and spent five months training at Fort Rucker in Alabama. He also continued to fly, logging over four thousand hours. He often flew his plane to Payson with another physician to help the small city out, as the medical clinic had no physician. Jack developed expertise in flying the Piper Apache, the Piper Comanche, the Piper Tripacer and the Aeronca Champ. As his children left home and married, he soon experienced the joys of becoming a grandparent. His grandchildren soon became familiar with the airports in the Phoenix area, as this was Jack's favorite way of eating breakfast. For a special breakfast treat, Jack enjoyed flying into a beautiful area near the Red Rocks of Sedona and landing at a small airport there that has a great restaurant to enjoy breakfast at while watching the planes take off or land.

During this time, he became close friends to another physician Aaron Bornstein who traveled with Jack to a continuing education medical seminar in Russia. The flight turned out to be amusing; in one Russia plane, dinner was a whole chicken dropped on the tray in a greasy bag, pinfeathers still attached. Their tours of the hospitals and the technology available determined Russia to be far below the standards of the United States. The average life span of a Russian man is 60 years old so most do not live long enough to collect a pension.

Russia has universal health care in that every citizen is entitled to free treatment but enormous problems have developed. Patients are in run down hospitals where staff may not provide enough attention and providers demand payments that force patients to scramble to pay fees up front to get proper emergency treatment. While all Russian citizens have "standardized" medical insurance, consumers who are more affluent pay privately and buy extra insurance to obtain proper medical care.

In the United States, the enormous advances in technology in pharmaceuticals and diagnostic equipment kept the insurance companies involved with any payment system focused on cost containment. Financial concerns to maximize profit were a high priority for the insurance company and this drive for cost containment became evident in the attitudes of providers, nurses and health care facilities including for-profit hospitals and unfortunately not-for-profit as well. Not-for-profit hospitals have the advantage of a tax exemption status in exchange for the provision of providing uncompensated healthcare to the public, but Jack saw charity transforming to competition. The complex structure of the not-for-profit hospitals makes it difficult to determine where these hospitals are failing in their obligations to their community but Jack questioned the effectiveness of the tax subsidy as a mechanism to increase indigent healthcare.

As managed care forced family practice providers to work for HMOs, Jack was busy expanding his practice in military medicine. He was the Flight Surgeon for the Arizona Army National Guard for 14 years. During this time helicopters in use at the Guard were the "Huey" an aircraft used in Vietnam from the early 1960s. Many of the pilots at the Guard who Jack worked with were Vietnam veterans and he was able to hear first hand descriptions of the use of these helicopters in that war. Originally, the Huey was used for transporting troops into strategic positions and then evacuating the wounded. Soon they were adapted and used as armed assault aircraft in order to protect the "grunts" or troops on the ground in combat. Jack soon became very familiar with soldiers who had post-traumatic stress disorder known as PTSD. Jack had to ground any pilot who had a medical or emotional condition that would affect his ability to fly.

Jack was able to work during his years as flight surgeon with his son Patrick who was an instructor pilot in the Huey. He also worked with his fourth son, Francis Xavier McCarville. Frank joined the Arizona Army National Guard in 1984 and spent time training in Fort Rucker Alabama in flight operations. He worked as an Active Duty National Guard (AGR) assigned to Operation Support Airlift with a C-12 aircraft that flies staff officers and higher officials who come into the Arizona area. Frank was deployed to Kuwait in support of Operation Iraqi Freedom in 2004. He was deployed again in October of 2008 to Baghdad, Iraq to help coordinate flights there. Jack is able to enjoy the advances of communication and keeps in contact with his son in Iraq with daily email. Frank has a favorite story about his father. When he asked him to pin his rank on during his promotion ceremony Jack pinned his rank on his collar sideways.

Jack enjoyed a heavier weight visiting all the wonderful new restaurants in the city of Phoenix but he knew weight gain had a relationship to the causes of Type II diabetes.

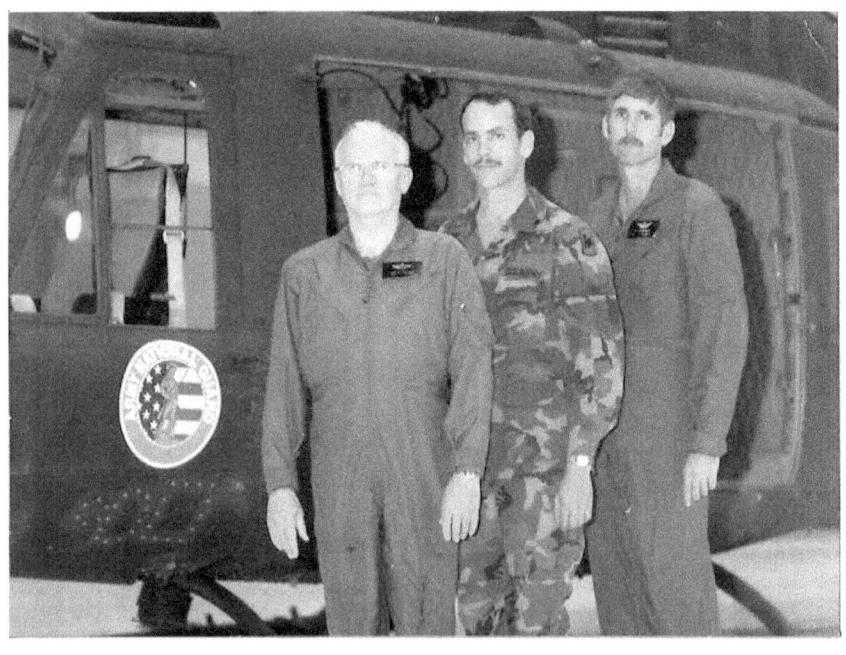

Jack and sons Francis Xavier and Patrick John at the Arizona Army National Guard

Researchers have traveled to Arizona to study the Pima Indians on the Gila Indian Reservation where Ira Hayes had lived. The Pima have one of the highest rates of diabetes in the world. Studies reveal a genetic cause for diabetes - the "thrifty gene" theory. In primitive times, Native Americans suffered times of near starvation, usually during the winter months. Evolution designed a gene to prompt the fat cell to develop more rapidly with the ingestion of food during abundant times to help carry the body through a period of starvation. This is an important gene to have if food is not available but now the gene is not necessary for survival. Jack confirmed this research when he traveled to Columbia University Medical Center in New York and learned about the work at the Naomi Berrie Diabetes Center. Laboratory studies on mice revealed that an abundant supply of food causes a single fat cell in the adipose tissue to enlarge. Once the fat cell reaches a certain size, the mitochondria, which contains genetic material and is responsible for cell metabolism, produces a super oxide rather than oxygen. Under the microscope the abnormal mitochondria in the fat cell appears black; hence the term "brown fat." This type of fat in a person especially in the abdominal area appears to have a relationship to an increased incidence of diabetes mellitus, hypertension, and hyperlipidemia, currently known as the metabolic syndrome.

Jack was concerned when he suddenly noticed he was urinating more frequently and was thirsty all the time. He was an avid mountain climber, exercised daily, and for a few weeks had felt the summer heat and his exercise schedule was taking its toll. He scheduled himself for a flight physical as he flew many different aircraft himself and was due to renew his license. He sat in shocked silence when the physician told him his blood work had revealed that he had diabetes. The diagnosis of diabetes mellitus cost him dearly. He now had to retire from the Army and his work as the Flight Surgeon, but even worse, he was not qualified to pilot a plane. Although he never did fly a plane after that day, he is often a passenger.

When he attended a medical seminar in Hawaii and was sitting in the plane for hours, he realized that he is most at home in the air. On that trip, the clock reached a minute after midnight and he had a birthday in the air at 30,000 feet over the Pacific Ocean.

After Jack's diagnoses of diabetes, he retired as a Colonel from the Arizona Army National Guard and devoted his entire practice to aviation as a FAA Medical Examiner and moved his office near Sky Harbor airport. He became a patient of Daniel Murphy who was a physician from Canada, another country with universal health care. They often discussed the subject of universal health care coverage, which dominated the headlines of the 2008 presidential election. The democrats appear to propose a variety of methods to cover the uninsured. They require the unemployed or self-employed to purchase their own health insurance and require employers to provide health insurance. Others would be included in

Medicaid or other government programs. Republicans will not expand the government health care programs as much; they tend to promote greater incentives for consumers to purchase their own healthcare coverage in a competitive marketplace. Presently almost 47 million Americans do not have health insurance, or about 16% of our population. Our new President Obama will have to deal with increasing unemployment and due to the poor economic state of the country; this number will continue to increase.

Most people Jack talked to believe they have a right to have universal healthcare provided by the government. The Indian Health Service, Medicare, Medicaid and the military are the closest examples of what universal health care coverage is in our country. However, this insurance is limited to certain populations. The problems and inefficiencies of Medicare will no doubt repeat themselves with universal health care and restrict individual liberties. Jack realizes with his experiences in his own practice as a physician that healthcare is subject to market forces. It is necessary to promote efficiency, ensure fairness, recognize the rights of third parties and preserve freedom and individual liberties. Jack's experience with his travels to Russia and his knowledge about the Canadian system from his friend Dr. Murphy gives him serious reservations about universal healthcare.

Ireland has had a socialized universal health care plan since 2005. The people of Ireland have shown satisfaction of the plan to be high in some surveys. However, the population of Ireland is small and unique. The plan resembles a four-leaf clover. Administration is divided into north, south, east and west under one single national entity called the Health Service Executive. Each section has offices locally where fees are collected or paid out; funds are obtained by general taxation. Free care is provided for all children and maternity patients, the elderly over 70 years of age, people with chronic diseases and anyone on welfare. This population receives free eye exams, hearing aids, eye care and dental care. The percentage of Ireland that qualifies for this free care is about 30%, certified with a medical card. The rest of the population has co pays for their services, set according to income.

Fortunately, in Ireland, visits to an emergency room with a referral from a family doctor are free and technologies such as X-Rays are free. In addition to universal health care, private health insurance is available to anyone who wishes additional coverage. This insurance is regulated and by law, all premiums are the same and no one can be refused. The low prices encourage competition among the insurance companies. Children and students and other low-income groups receive a 50% discount, about 60% of the population purchases this additional insurance. General practitioners make house calls in Ireland and do not charge those too poor to pay. Advocating universal healthcare on a political level is desirable, as no normal person would oppose health insurance for children. Hazards emerge when consumers over consume and raise costs for others, increasing co-pays, deductibles and reducing the number of covered procedures and the quality of healthcare. Medicare determined Congress failed to realize how the lowering of reimbursement rates to providers would have them respond by reducing the availability of medical services. Controlling costs by rationing healthcare reduces quality and healthcare itself becomes a scarce good.

Jack still devotes his entire practice to aviation medicine as an FAA Medical Examiner in Phoenix. It would be safe to say that the majority of airline pilots know who he is and many have their current medical licenses in their wallet with his signature. Pilots must have a pilot's license but he or she must also have their health certified by a medical exam every 6 to 12 months. Jack's office manager, Kathleen Mizanin, has worked for him for over 23 years. Their worst day together was when they received a call from the FAA informing them that records showed a 9/11 terrorist who had a pilot's license had been to Jack's office and obtained a medical license. Jack had examined a pilot who was a terrorist who trained those who flew the planes into the Twin Towers. This information was public and Kathleen had to battle many reporters who wanted information about the terrorist who had been to Jack's office. Homeland security is now more involved with the ability of pilots to obtain a pilot's license.

Jack attends FAA Medical Examiner seminars the most recent was in 2008, an international conference in Germany to review how other countries certify their pilots. Some countries require a two day exam. Waivers are important for pilots with special medical conditions that are still capable of flying and Jack was the first physician to obtain a waiver for a medical license for a pilot who had a melanoma. Although Jack could obtain waivers for pilots, on rare occasions the FAA instructed Jack to ground pilots for drug and alcohol problems or PTSD.

The growing number of children caused Jack to have a contractor come into his home and remodel the garage into a large bedroom for the five boys. When Jack and Marge had their eighth child, Marge's sister Arlene gave birth to her eleventh child. Years later Arlene walked out to the kitchen one morning and her husband John was slumped over the table, dead from a stroke. Arlene was now a mother to eleven children without a father. As the years went by, Jack and Marge slowly suffered through a divorce. Jack never imagined the Irish Catholic disapproval he would receive from his family in Iowa. Although Marge never remarried, Jack raised Irish eyebrows in Iowa again when he married a British girl, Patricia Oakley. They met while ballroom dancing and Jack enjoyed her stories of England as she described her life as a teenager watching dogfights over London with the Spitfire and the Messerschmitt. She suffered the terror of bombers coming in the dark of night during the Battle of Britain, which lasted for nine months. She then became very familiar with buzz bombs and V2 rockets. Jack thought she was very brave. Everyone learned how brave she was when she became a paraplegic after a car accident. Jack and his family grew to admire and respect the fact that she never complains about her condition.

After their divorce, Marge wanted to downsize and move to a condominium. Like his great great grandfather Dennis Daniel in Willow Springs, Jack was proud of the house he had built in Phoenix. He did not have the heart to sell the large custom home. His children were very happy when Jack moved into the old house with his second wife Patricia after having the house constructed to be wheelchair accessible for her. Jack's entire family, his children, grandchildren and great grandchildren including Marge, meet there to celebrate every holiday.

Father Charles, the brother of Marge and Arlene, keeps in close contact with his Arizona family. For the anniversary of his 25th year in the priesthood, Father Charles flew his two sisters, Marge and Arlene and every niece and nephew living in Arizona back for a reunion in Iowa. These children were able to visit the homes their parents grew up in, visit the various cemeteries and churches important to their families, and meet their Iowa cousins. Jack's mother Catherine died later on December 20, 1988 of heart failure.

Francis and Jack became close after her death when Jack made a special visit to Iowa with his daughter Michelle. On that trip, while sitting together in the evening after dinner, Francis discussed the Irish family tree. Michelle began to take notes on a yellow legal pad she still has today. She admired how strong her grandfather Francis was and could not help but marvel at how brilliant blue his eyes were. Michelle and Jack listened together for hours to his stories about the family history. When Francis spoke of Thomas I and II, Dennis Daniel and son Dennis Michael to Jack and Michelle, they became alive again. After Francis was finished talking about the family, he walked Michelle to her bedroom and kissed her goodnight. She thought about her grandfather that night and his avid interest in her writing notes while he was talking.

Francis made a special effort to visit Jack when Michelle's first child, Rachel Brianna Kennedy was born on March 22, 1990. Francis died soon after on October 14, 1990 in Moorland, Iowa from a stroke.

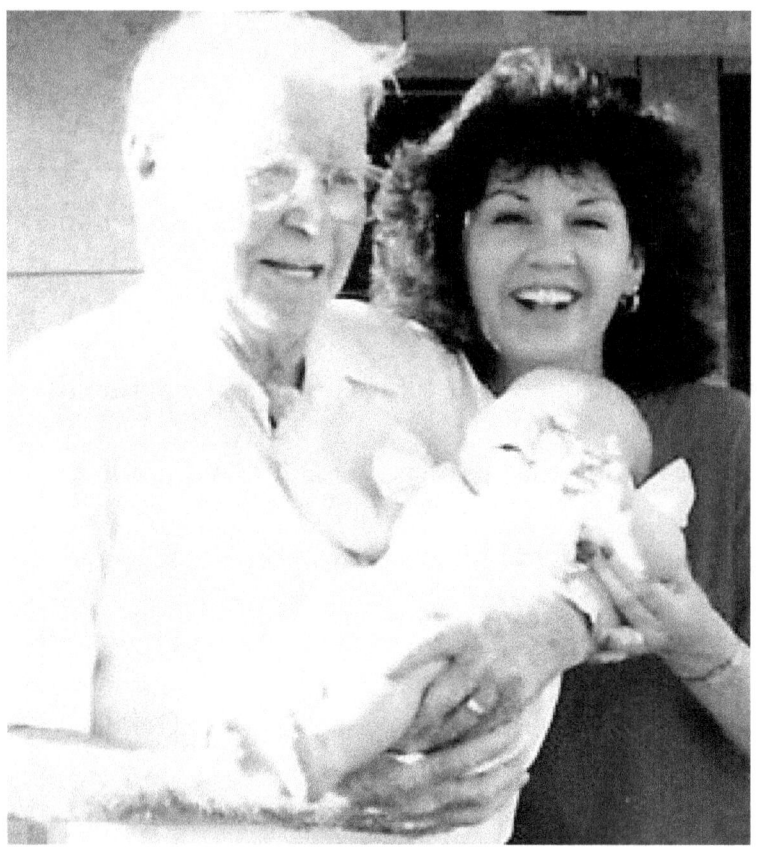

Francis McCarville, Rachel Brianna Kennedy and Mary Michele McCarville, 1990

Because of the long-term effects of diabetes, Jack developed high cholesterol and had difficulty controlling it. While at his grandson Tommy Gladden's birthday party, he noticed both his arms and elbows were sore. He made sure he enjoyed the chocolate birthday cake before he left the party and drove to his office. He noticed he was having anxiety and his pain continued in both arms so he performed an EKG on himself. He stood up in shock when he read the EKG; he was having a heart attack. When he arrived at the emergency room at the hospital, he handed the EKG over to the physician and his treatment started immediately. He eventually had to have heart bypass surgery. He had his surgery at the hospital where he had delivered his first baby and where most of his eight children were born. This was Saint Josephs' Hospital in Phoenix. He was able to witness, as a patient, the changes in cardiac care. Jack did not have the Sisters at Saint Joseph's supervising his care. They are not there anymore. Instead, besides his heart surgeon, Jack had a hospitalist caring for him while he was in the hospital. Hospitalists are physicians with a background in internal medicine who communicate with the primary physicians but manage the care of the patient while in the hospital. This can be an advantage for the patient as these physicians work at the hospital full time and are familiar with the system. Jack realized that a hospitalist could make a lucrative income as they charge for each patient's care and can see a great deal of patients. In addition to the skill and expertise of his physicians, Jack had technology. When Jack was a child, heart attack patients rested in bedrooms with no real treatment available.

After Jack recovered from surgery, he firmly believes in the benefits of his trips to the gym and the new goal for prevention in medicine. Efforts to determine how to prevent disease and stay healthy are being made in new and unusual ways and insurance companies in some areas are now covering complementary medicine. Complementary medicine, traditional medicine philosophy and alternative medicine all have different characteristics. The traditional medicine philosophy is our western medicine, which is a scientifically proven method for treating medical conditions, where physicians practice and insurance companies pay. Complementary medicine, which Jack observed with Native Americans, can be used along with mainstream medical care. Smoking a pipe for prayer or having a medicine man perform a ceremony with the patient can be used with regular western medical care. An insurance company does not pay for these practices but a few others are. Acupuncture can be billed and paid for by insurance such as Blue Cross Blue Shield and Medicare. Other widely accepted methods of complementary medicine can be covered such as chiropractic therapy. Complementary medicine is accepted by the providers of the patient and recommended if it has developed into the mainstream of medicine or been proven to be effective. These methods can improve the quality of life; some other examples are aromatherapy and massage.

Alternative medicine is used without conventional treatment and is an unproven method. When Jack was in general practice, some of his patients in the terminal stages of cancer would turn to alternative medicine in a desperate hope to stay alive. Alternative medicine provides great hope especially in terminal states, but fraud has been a problem in this area. The interruption of regular medical care can advance a disease state and put a patient in the hands of people who have no credentials. However, alternative methods may work and need to be investigated. One of the ways to discover if these alternative methods work is by clinical trials. Wellness centers are starting to enter the preventive market. Employers, managed care plans and insurance companies are promoting prevention, which helps with cost effectiveness. Jack's trips to the gym have been so important to his health he believes medical insurance should pay for gym memberships. Medicare is covering services that are more preventive and this will prevent disease and decrease spending. The epidemic in obesity and diabetes can be managed more effectively with prevention and education.

One of the biggest challenges the healthcare market faces in the United States is a shortage of staff in the industry. The shortage is in nursing, pharmacy, primary care disciplines and many others. The causes of the shortage vary and include medical staff leaving their profession due to workplace dissatisfaction or fears of malpractice resulting from the increases of patient to staff ratios. Primary care providers suffer a loss in autonomy due to managed care in addition to the rising cost of malpractice insurance. In the nursing profession, some leave jobs in hospital staffing to further their education and career by becoming a physician assistant. Additional reasons for the healthcare shortage include poor pay scales for long or undesirable hours, insurance benefit conflicts, an aging healthcare workforce and universities restricting program enrollments to students interested in various healthcare fields due to a shortage of classroom space and instructors. Some married couples who both happen to be doctors are cutting back their hours in the workforce due to fears of increased taxes.

As technology and advances in computers continue, healthcare will become a paperless system. The electronic health record (EHR) will decrease administration and documentation costs. Telemedicine will help consumers obtain healthcare and increase access to healthcare to everyone - everywhere. Arizona has one of the most advanced telemedicine networks in the United States, developed by the University of Arizona, even on remote Indian reservations. Telemedicine may be one answer to the shortage of providers in healthcare.

Jack believes everyone has a right to have access to quality healthcare at an affordable price. He recently questioned other medical professionals on what they thought was going to happen to the future of healthcare now that we have a new president in office in 2009. They all agree most likely, universal healthcare or not, technology will influence the marketplace dynamics. However, when Jack considers the future of healthcare he considers his ancestor Dennis Daniel who left Ireland to come to America, for freedom. Freedom is a paramount issue in healthcare when making laws and policies. Consumers have a right and responsibility to make informed decisions on their healthcare and healthcare options should be available. Healthcare should be based on our rights to freedom as Americans, not on an inability in the production of healthcare or on the lack of resources. As Jack continues to practice as a First Class FAA Medical Examiner in Phoenix, Arizona in 2009, he looks back at the many changes in healthcare that have happened during his career in medicine. Sometimes, we may have to look into the past to see the future.

About the Author

Mary Michele McCarville, known as Michelle, is the second child of John and Margaret McCarville out of their family of eight. Jack and Marge chose her name in honor of St. Michael when she was born on the Feast of the Guardian Angels, October 2. She worked with her father as an LPN before obtaining her BS in Pharmacy from the University of Arizona in 1984 and received her MHA in 2008 from the University of Phoenix. She has worked as a pharmacist for various Native Americans tribes in Arizona for over 25 years. Mary Michele has two children, Rachel Brianna Kennedy from a previous marriage to Kirk Allen Kennedy, and Thomas Michael Gladden. Both of her children have inherited Jack's trait of loving to ride horses. Michelle is married to Thomas Eugene Gladden who retired from the Army after sustaining an injury while deployed to Afghanistan in Operation Enduring Freedom. Michelle is active in supporting deployed soldiers from the Arizona Army National Guard.

www.ingramcontent.com/pod-product-compliance
Lightning Source LLC
Chambersburg PA
CBHW051643170526
45167CB00001B/305